FRENCH WOMEN FOR ALL SEASONS

ALSO BY MIREILLE GUILIANO

French Women Don't Get Fat

French Women

FOR ALL SEASONS

A Year of Secrets, Recipes, & Pleasure

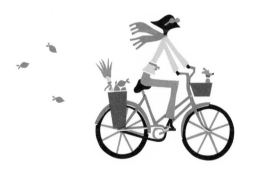

MIREILLE GUILIANO

RANDOM HOUSE CANADA

LIBRARY AND ARCHIVES CANADA CATALOGUING IN PUBLICATION
Guiliano, Mireille, [date]
French women for all seasons : a year of secrets, recipes & pleasure / Mireille Guiliano.
ISBN-13: 978-0-679-31489-9
ISBN-10: 0-679-31489-X
1. Cookery, French. 2. Food habits—France. 3. Food—Psychological aspects.
4. Women—Health and hygiene--France. I. Title.
RM222.2.G83 2006   641.5944   C2006-903006-5

First Edition

Printed and bound in the United States of America

10 9 8 7 6 5 4 3 2 1

Live in each season as it passes; breathe the air, drink the drink, taste the fruit, and resign yourself to the influences of each. Let them be your only diet drink and botanical medicines.

—*Henry David Thoreau*

CONTENTS

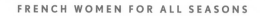

FRENCH WOMEN FOR ALL SEASONS

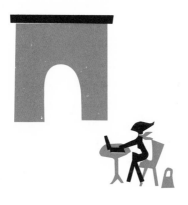

"It was the best of times, it was the worst of times." Thus Charles Dickens began his *Tale of Two Cities* a century and a half ago. The cities he imagined were Paris and London. The countries he was contrasting were revolutionary France and late-eighteenth-century England. Two opposing worlds, two points of view. And two divergent destinies. When I wrote *French Women Don't Get Fat,* I had in mind two disparate worlds of eating: the French and the American. Also, to a lesser extent, two cities, Paris and New York. What I did not realize at the time was that I was in fact writing a tale of two global cultures increasingly without borders. For better and worse, where you live no longer dictates how you eat. It's up to you.

Even in our ever more complex world, it is still possible

to have our cake and eat it too, to enjoy our days to the fullest in many ways while embracing a time-tested, back-to-basics approach to life—one filled with quality, sensitivity, seasonal foods, and pleasure. I don't want to live in the past, but I *do* want to learn from it, and I believe that the culture of moderation, painstaking attention to taste, and healthy eating and living that I absorbed growing up in France can be adapted to today's world and pursued just about anywhere. This is not to say I don't understand or appreciate firsthand the challenges women these days face: the pressures of too much to do in too little time, of mega portions and industrially produced food often eaten on the run.

For a long time, this clash of cultural and lifestyle perspectives and outcomes took shape in my mind as a contrast between on the one hand fundamental elements of French culture and on the other behaviors I learned in America. But with the appearance of *French Women Don't Get Fat* in language after language, I have come to understand that what I thought of as a national divide is really only an emblem for a conflict of two world orders. While I certainly don't think I have all the solutions to this conflict, or any highly specialized expertise—I try not to take myself too seriously—I still have more experiences and secrets (and many more recipes and weekly menus) to share that will help people enjoy a better quality of life—and almost certainly lose weight.

Last fall a French reporter followed me through the Union Square Greenmarket in New York, where we encountered a class of eight-year-olds with their teacher. The kids were participating in a program called Spoons Across America, a not-for-profit organization dedicated to educating children, teachers, and families about the benefits of healthy eating and the value of supporting local farmers and sharing meals around the family table. As it was fall, apples of many varieties were abundantly available. But when the reporter, half kidding, picked one up and asked a little boy what it was, the child drew a blank. Forget the variety; he did not know it was an apple. This city kid had apparently never seen one in real life. It gives one pause. I would bet, though, that he could recognize the packaged apple pie at the McDonald's just opposite the greenmarket.

The world where I grew up—and my experience of apples—in Alsace-Lorraine could not have been farther from this little boy's in New York City. As I recall it, all our neighbors had at least one fruit tree, and we had numerous apple trees in our garden. Come apple-picking time, my job was to place the different varieties we grew into little flat crates called *cagettes*, which we put into the cold cellar for winter storage— a centuries-old practice now mostly gone. What sweet and glorious aromas filled that cellar when I deposited all those baskets! (Tellingly, in French the word for smell, *sentir*, also means feel.) Today I recall the apple smell even more powerfully than the old footage of that autumn ritual I carry around in my head. And, of course, the harvest meant my mother would once again make an apple pie, *une tarte aux pommes alsacienne*.

In our garden we also had bushes of *groseilles*, tart red currants that are a regional specialty. My mother and I loved to make pies with these tiny berries. The season for red currants is short, and we quickly made jam *(confiture)* or jelly *(gelée)* or pies, and sometimes a sauce *(coulis)*. And oh, how we looked forward to this once-a-year treat, which somehow exemplifies for me the French woman's psychological pleasure in food. It is the anticipation and joy that we gain from a pleasure we cannot take for granted and know we will soon lose. Tasting such seasonal bounty heightens our awareness of what we put into our mouths and contrasts with routine, mindless eating that provides little pleasure and often unwanted pounds.

These days, an image I carry around with me is of two airports. It's fitting, since airports are now the crossroads of the world, the most common interface of one culture with another. At O'Hare International, in Chicago, on the way to an appearance on the *Oprah* show, I witnessed a surreal spectacle I wish I had videotaped. People all around me in the terminal were gulping down hamburgers, fries, and pizza and knocking back big tubs of soda or coffee as they tapped away on their laptops, talked on cell phones, and flipped through newspapers. Most remarkable: it was 10 a.m. Why were they even eating? I asked myself. Breakfast? Early lunch? Or just a way to pass the time? It looked more like stuffing than eating, actually. And most of the people I saw were significantly overweight. Plus, I could not detect pleasure on a single face. On my way back to New York, it was equally disturbing to see the airport bars doing a brisk business at 3 p.m. Here and there, however, one could spot people not of this place: American abstainers from the madness? Or perhaps visitors just passing through? Anyway, these people reminded me of the French approach.

The airport–cum–food court may be a sign of the times, but not quite yet in France. At Charles de Gaulle (or Roissy, as the French call it), the busiest hub on the Continent, when French people eat, they still generally sit down with a knife and fork at enclosed cafeterias or restaurants. There are small stand-up bars for those who want a quick croissant or perhaps a *jambon beurre* and a cup of coffee. But have you seen a typical French cup of coffee? Three sips, four max. No frappuccino gargantuoso con lateria or whatever (though Starbucks has followed McDonald's as a global brand). In France, if you want milk, you order a *crème* or even a *grand crème*—add a few more sips. The airports may still reflect the traditional differences, for the most part, but they also show that infiltration is taking place in both directions. Things in France aren't yet set up to accommodate the contemporary culture of excess, but where there's a will, there's a way: in the odd corner you do find people engaging in alien habits, with two sandwiches, an iPod, and a magazine feeding them all at once. But in France they are the exception; in America they rule.

Ever since that day in Chicago, whenever I see such scenes, I think of a quote by Brillat-Savarin, the eighteenth-century "modern" gastronome, well known for his writings and meditations on the physiology of taste and for his famous dictum "We are what we eat." But he also wrote even more revealingly: "The destiny of a nation depends on how it feeds itself."

Even Paris, famed as the world capital of slender women, isn't immune to the growing culture of excess and the global breakdown in traditional ways of eating. Some readers have gone so far as to send me "gotcha" letters informing me that, while in France, they actually saw a fat French woman! *Vraiment*. I never said they don't exist. While the vast majority are not fat, there is indeed an—*excusez-moi!*—growing minority of the *bouboule* (overweight and dumpy), many of whom are not far from becoming obese. How could it be? Fast-food chains arrived years ago on the boulevard Saint-Germain and the Champs-Élysées. French women are not immune to the primal urges for the sweet and salty that make fast food appealing. But even more important, they are not exempt from the pressures of living and working in a globalized world that erodes traditional local values and speeds up the pace of life, leaving less time for savoring food as our parents did. As eating becomes less and less a family affair, mothers and fathers neglect to teach their children the right way to eat. Bad habits rush to fill the void. (There's even a public service ad campaign in France with the slogan *L'obésité Tue*, "Obesity kills.") Make no mistake: overeating is an approaching global epidemic (already arrived in many countries). Unless we get our act together, in one generation the French will be as dangerously overweight as many Americans and other nationalities and will fit perfectly into a contemporary airport movie.

If the threat were not real, *French Women Don't Get Fat* would have been a curiosity instead of a phenomenon when it was published in France in 2005. My native land, it seemed, wanted to be reminded of its own traditional habits almost as much as my adoptive homeland wanted to be introduced to them. In the twenty-first century, we can no longer expect to receive lifestyle as an inheritance; it has become a matter of active choice. There is no *cordon sanitaire* to keep Pizza Hut Poppers out of France.

On the other hand, there is also virtually nothing barring you from importing what is beneficial in the classic French lifestyle and finding ways of making it work where you live. Long ago, I made the connection that a serious interest in food, this pillar of the French lifestyle, is the main reason that, overwhelmingly and by tradition, French women don't get fat. My first book was addressed to the untold legions of diet victims, people all over the world, whom I urged to reject the twin hoaxes of (1) deprivation is the key to weight loss and (2) indulgence is to blame for weight gain. Pleasure has proved to be the most powerful and lasting motivation, even more compelling than the dream of dropping a dress size. Actually it was just common sense reborn: if we can all harness the pleasure principle, we can lose weight, as French women have done for generations. All we need is to learn a sense of proportion and cultivate our appreciation of taste. Do that and we should never feel deprived. I asked for a commitment of months, not weeks. But the promise in return was results that last—no yo-yoing (the pitfall of any quick-fix diet). My aim was to lead people to becoming effortlessly slender beings, alert and devoted to pleasure. I am hardly a champion of France in all things, just in some. And it's not out of some precious snobbery that I reject many of the things on supermarket shelves. When foods are bursting with natural taste—as opposed to being artificially flavored, laden with fat and salt, or just plain tasteless—the experience of eating them is more satisfying, and we can content ourselves with less. And so, when French women exult over some perfectly ripe melon, they are making a spectacle not just of themselves but of their capacity to register real degrees of difference—a talent nurtured by a culture in which things are harvested in season and bought fresh. This capacity, more than anything else, is their secret weapon in not getting fat. The pleasure of quality more than offsets the temptation of unlimited quantity.

French DNA is not necessary for the experience. French

women don't have thousands of extra little taste receptors that allow them to distinguish Jacques Torres's chocolates from Hershey's Kisses. They do, however, have a lifetime of exposure to and cultivated appreciation of the good stuff. This is something we can all develop. Helping to cultivate that knack—which requires an awareness of what each season has to offer—and thereby learn to reap all the invigorating benefits is one of my main purposes in writing this book.

Cost? Yes, as I've admitted, better things generally—though not always—cost more. But I am not asking readers to buy a ticket to the French Riviera. Many of the pleasures I suggest are inexpensive, from walking or bicycling to avoiding built-in transportation costs by buying local produce in season. The French do spend more per capita on food than, for instance, Americans or the British. But by eating better, you eat less. And the French have a lower per capita income to begin with. If it's a matter of your health, body image, and peace of mind, isn't it worth digging a little deeper? Everyone blows money on something, usually something less important than food. It's a question of conditioning and priorities—of which you may find you share more with the French than you realized.

Quality exists on the palate of the person, who must teach herself to distinguish it. Education is crucial. People need to understand what they are putting in their bodies. What are the consequences of drinking eight or ten ounces of orange juice in the morning? Even something as simple as bottled water requires attention. All bottled waters are not created equal. Read the label. Some of the best-selling brands have high levels of sodium, which people with high blood pressure or heart disease should avoid, and many mineral-rich waters have high calcium levels, which should be a red alert to those susceptible to kidney stones.

Cooking is also education: it raises your awareness of what you are feeding your body and when, sharpens your taste buds, and can help you develop the sort of relationship with food that inhibits overeating. Anybody can learn to cook. (Involving children in cooking and taking them food shopping in a market to see real ingredients and buy fresh can make a huge difference in their lives.) Cooking doesn't have to be difficult or time-consuming when the ingredients are fresh and good—the best preparations are the simplest. The recipes in this book overwhelmingly adhere to my philosophy of pure and simple, and always pleasure. (Once in a while, easy and simple is not the goal, though pleasure still is. Who doesn't enjoy ordering something in a restaurant that took someone else hours and hours to prepare?)

Of course, quality of life, French or otherwise, requires more than good food. The joy of living is in direct proportion to how much pleasure you know how to derive from *every* aspect of living. As I will describe, the French lifestyle offers examples of delicious experience beyond just the gastronomic. Everything from how we move to how we groom ourselves to how we greet each day has the potential for unlocking pleasure and making life feel fuller. There is, after all, more to life than not getting fat.

I have heard amazing stories *(merci beaucoup)* of successful self-transformation, changes of hearts and minds, as well as bodies, inspired by *French Women Don't Get Fat.* Voilà, the secret of pleasure in a nutshell: Change the way you think, and the way you eat will follow. Change the way you eat, and the pounds will take care of themselves. Conversely, let a diet book dictate how, what, where, and when you eat, and you will learn nothing, only postpone the inevitable relapse. In my first book I laid out the basics for a do-it-yourself turnaround, a path to weight loss and a happy equilibrium, that weight at which one feels *bien dans sa peau* (comfortable in one's skin). Now we proceed *peu à peu* (little by little), so that you are reborn for life, not just for the bikini season.

This new book is a guide to a deeper understanding of the basics I presented in the first. It is also a source of suggestions to take you through one year, and years to come of continually inventing and embracing pleasurable experience—the key to the good life as the French enjoy it. As always, I provide not templates but food for thought: I'll let you in on secrets of my own and of other French women, with tips, recipes, and menus (as well as insights on wine and cheese, *bien sûr*), but what you make of it is uniquely your own.

Here, then, is a continuation of the French lessons we began in *French Women Don't Get Fat*, in things my family and the savior of my youth, Dr. Miracle, taught me. I am perpetually adapting them to suit our busy lives. Nothing here, taken as always in moderation, will make you fat, but the express aim is rounding out your life (as opposed to your bottom). It is about embracing the seasons and seasonality and making eating and savoring life a more intense experience. It's learning the way to find pleasure in all things. I offer a new framework in which to contemplate some of the timeless principles of French women, as well as new ideas, the goal being to promote a more holistic approach to living. You're bound to pick up slimming pointers, but if your immediate concern is weight loss, why not start with the first book in order to achieve your point of stable equilibrium (a healthy weight that satisfies you)? While making no claims to literary genius, I do know that you can't enjoy Proust until you have made the time commitment and picked up sufficient vocabulary and grammar.

In *French Women Don't Get Fat* I introduced readers to the basic elements of joie de vivre; here we take up *l'art de vivre,* the finer points of living to the fullest. It may be that after this next level you'll be able to teach some French women a thing or two. In the late nineteenth century, American painters came to Barbizon to learn about art from the world's undisputed masters. A generation or so later it was the French painters seeking to learn from the Americans. As long as the lamp of French women remains lit, it hardly matters what nationality is holding it aloft. This is no more a tale of two cities.

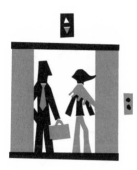

I

"J'ai oublié de vous dire" ("I forgot to tell you") was an expression of my mother's that I remember from a very young age. It seemed *Mamie* was always forgetting to tell you something important she had remembered only after you had left the room or hung up the phone. For instance: "Oh, and I forgot to tell you, if you don't beat your egg whites to firm peaks, your soufflé will collapse!"

Before my first book was launched in France, a Parisian friend had a dinner party with French ladies, some of whom had read the English version, eager to know what beans I had spilled. One of them, Michèle, who hadn't read a word, pressed me to declare what I had written. But before I could say anything, Claudette, another guest, said with mischievous nonchalance, "Oh, she has told them absolutely everything about how we eat without getting fat!" I laughed, a bit uneasy to see Michèle getting quite *énervée* (agitated). Finally she said, "How dare you give away OUR secrets to the world?" I am not making this up, and it wasn't a totally isolated incident in the company of French women. "We are all in this together," I said. "I was only trying to help a few troubled souls." Nothing would calm her down until I muttered, "Don't worry, *j'ai oublié de leur dire* [I forgot to tell them]. . . . I have not given away *all* our secrets." I didn't, however, take a vow of silence. . . .

PITFALLS OF THE ELEVATOR SPEECH

We live in a world far more complex than our parents' and grandparents', but in some ways our world is more superficial. People, my fellow New Yorkers not least, want short answers and quick solutions, and in their multitasking universe they can't spare the attention to think deeply or focus for too long on any one problem—even a problem as immediate as their own excess weight.

The elevator speech—a form invented and perfected in Manhattan—is the notion that in a world where time is money and attention spans are short, you have only thirty seconds to sell your new idea. Depending on the elevator, this is roughly equivalent to the time required to ride the car up ten floors, during which you are holding a decision maker captive. "If you can't get your idea across in a few sentences, you haven't refined your thinking"; so goes the prevailing business-speak. Well, I suppose that's true for many simple innovations, from double-sided tape (excellent invention) to multicolor umbrella hats (beats me). Some ideas, even good ones, really need only thirty seconds.

There are, however, somewhat more involved propositions that don't lend themselves to this format. What thirty-second version of a political philosophy would you subscribe to? Diets, on the other hand, being consumer products, must toe the line of brevity. For instance, "It's all about carb restriction" or "It's not what you eat but when you eat it." People wanted me to sum up in thirty seconds my own program for life, which I have always presented as emphatically as I could as a nondiet with a holistic approach. The elevator synopsis of *French Women Don't Get Fat* includes mention of rediscovering the pleasures of eating and cooking. "Eat three meals a day; keep portions small; eat seasonal fruits and vegetables; drink lots of water; savor wine; walk more; and have occasional treats." But, that's so general it can apply to many books and is rightly called common sense. Reduced to a set of bullet points, the whole really is much less than the sum of its parts. A lifestyle, however, or way of life, is a set of behaviors by which you adopt lasting principles and embody certain values. No one point on its own, or even listed together, gives a complete picture, any more than a plot summary could give you a whole book. A book is a thing to be read and absorbed over time. By contrast, a diet is not a lifestyle (heaven forbid!) any more than a diet book (really just an instructional manual) is, properly speaking, a book to be savored and enjoyed.

To read a book is, at least for a time, to try on a different way of thinking, a way of seeing, and in this case, a way of eating, moving, and living. A complete turnaround in the way you eat, move, and live properly takes six months to a year. It's admittedly more of an investment of time than plugging numbers into a calorie chart—I may well have neglected to make clear in the first book the need for patience and perseverance. (Prescribing pleasures, not deprivations, I guess I assumed pleasures pay their own way—don't they?) Results, as many readers have reported, do come in direct proportion to application: the more you think about change, the more things you wind up changing; the more things you change, the better your whole life becomes. Sort of the opposite of the never-ending cycle of diets: a brief interval of unpleasantness in exchange for a brief respite from your woes. If you really want to drop a quick ten pounds just for a few weeks—I don't advise it—a diet, though never healthful, may serve you fine. But if you want to drop the weight permanently and enjoy life while keeping it off, keep on reading. This book promises deeper understanding of my philosophy and therefore even more pleasures, a level of mastery where weight management and other benefits become pretty much effortless.

But before we get into some lengthier chapter presentations, here are some afterthoughts, reaffirmations, and a few more secrets that "I forgot to tell you."

FRENCH WOMEN LIVE LONGER

A few years ago, the oldest person in the world died. She was 122 years old and lived in the south of France, in Arles, the big old town that passes for a city in Provence. Much about her life has been scrutinized and verified: she ate a traditional French-Mediterranean diet, local seasonal fruits and vegetables, olives, olive oil, a moderate amount of freshly killed meats and fowl, and fish. Her fat intake was mainly of good fat, though doubtless she enjoyed her cheeses and the occasional pat of butter. Eating locally grown produce, she would have ingested relatively little in the way of pesticides, pollutants, and preservatives and certainly no genetically modified foods. I don't know that she drank magical leek soup, but she surely ate leeks. She enjoyed a daily glass or two of the local wine, which is almost exclusively red; she also liked a taste of port before meals. She did not eat fast food. She did not eat good food quickly. She ate three meals a day at a pace suited to savoring them. Walking and bicycling were her primary means of transportation (the latter till age one hundred), and she lived by the clock of Provence, where deadlines exist in only the laxest sense and there are long midday breaks for lunch and perhaps a nap. (When my husband, Edward, and I are in Provence, we have three wall clocks. One is set to New York time, one to Paris time; the third is set to Provence time [literally the same as Paris's but not really]. We never added batteries to that clock as a reminder it never seems necessary to keep track of the local time exactly. Come to think of it, the New York clock is probably the most stressful thing we have in that house.)

Oh, and I forgot to mention, this long-lived woman was never fat.

We cannot all turn the clock back a century, move to Provence, and live the life of Jeanne Louise Calment, into our hundreds. To be honest, though a long life sounds good, I would not want to live hers. I like mine. But her example offers a great lesson—indeed, many lessons—from which any of us can profit. For although she was alone in the *Guinness*

Book of World Records, her life as a French woman of her generation was not atypical.

According to the World Health Organization, French
women have the highest life expectancy in the Western world
and, excluding Japan, the highest worldwide. Today a French
woman can expect to reach the age of 82.8. One of the reasons
is simple: despite alarming trends in the opposite direction,
French women overall still don't get fat. And the greatest risk
factors for mortality in the developed world are the diseases
associated with obesity. If she had been fat, Jeanne Louise
Calment could not have been riding her bike at age one hundred, even in the unlikely event that she had lived to see that
age.

Medical science has made remarkable strides in extending the human lifespan by successfully treating many in-
fectious agents and life-threatening cancers and managing
chronic conditions such as diabetes. But in those countries
where the benefits of modern medicine are most readily available, the lifestyle choices are often fighting against the benefits
of science.

Most of us would prefer not to be fat. But do we have the
time and the means to take as good care of ourselves as did
Jeanne Louise Calment? Our lives may in many ways be far
more complicated than the traditional French life, but it's well
to remember that all those French women living past eighty
today were born into the difficulties of the Depression and
survived the occupation of their country during the Second
World War and regular shortages of basic necessities. You
think you've got stress! It wasn't all picking cherries in the
Vaucluse for them either. The example of French women

teaches that good habits can help us endure stress and, if properly instilled, can be maintained under the most adverse circumstances. French women traditionally live, as the expression goes, *entre deux âges* (between two ages, or of ambiguous age). Your actual number of years upon the earth is one thing, but after a certain point it is the condition of your mind and body that will dictate your physical and mental age and, by extension, how you feel. (We are not like trees, whose cross sections reveal indisputable rings of truth.) Short-term, French women don't get fat. Consequently, long-term, French women stay young, living not just longer but better lives.

THE 50 PERCENT SOLUTION

If, as one critic commented on *French Women Don't Get Fat*, it's "all about portion size"—it's not, really, but *if*—then change is indeed a tall order. It's generally known that Americans on average eat 10 to 30 percent more than we need to every day. This is not such a surprising result of an increasingly knowledge-based economy, in which the jobs of many individuals involve sitting all day. It is simple deductive reasoning to connect this situation with the fact that Americans are also on average 30 percent above their ideal weight. It was a sixteenth-century Frenchman, Montaigne, who rightly observed that gluttony is the source of all our infirmities. In the land where there's honor in being able to eat the most hot dogs, what is one to do?

Portion control is more an art than a discipline, one grounded in a useful bit of self-deception. I have written about the power of incrementalism, cutting back portions over weeks and months as you introduce new variety. Though very simple, the method sometimes requires a scale and can be a bit too unstructured for some.

One trick I use to control my intake is to ask myself if I can live with half the amount being offered; indeed, will I be just as happy eating half as much? I put this approach into play in a variety of ways, from splitting a dessert with my husband to counting the number of pieces of bread I eat in a restaurant. (Bread is one of my "offenders," a food I'm particularly vulnerable to overeating, and I can mindlessly eat three or four slices if I don't pay attention.) I use this simple alternative regularly, especially when not sure about the "hidden" ingredients of what I've been served or when the portion I've been offered is obviously large. I eat half. Slowly, of course, chewing well. I then ask myself whether I'm content, and therefore whether continuing would be a matter of pleasure or merely routine.

Contentment with most foods, in terms of taste, is to be found in the first few bites. It's your brain that tells your stomach what's enough, not vice versa. After that, another psychological phenomenon kicks in: that of literally filling ourselves, which evolution perhaps favors as a hedge against starvation, making it a pleasant feeling (at least until you're totally bloated) and therefore a natural impulse.

Often I do continue eating, but I have only half of the half that's left. Then, after pausing, I consider half of what's left again. Edward calls this my Zeno's Paradox of portion control. To paraphrase the ancient principle, if you continue eating only half of what's on your plate each time, you will never eat the whole thing. That's a theoretical explanation. I'm content to call it the 50 Percent Solution and think more practically about why it works. The act of stopping and reflecting slows down consumption, allowing the brain to catch up with the stomach and release the hormone that tells us, "Mmm, that was good, but I've had enough." Contentment is largely a matter of the clock—not just how much you ingest but also what you've eaten during a given interval.

If you implement the 50 Percent Solution routinely, your sense of a satisfying portion is bound to shrink. I've been doing it so long it even works on a banana.

Bananas are a welcome staple, available year-round since they grow in tropical climes not subject to the seasons of our temperate zone. Certainly in winter they fill out the relative dearth of fresh fruit. And they are good for you: low in saturated fat, cholesterol, and sodium and a good source of dietary fiber, vitamin C, potassium, manganese, and vitamin B_6. Most of their calories, though, come from sugars, which increase with ripeness, so they are a potential offender and must be eaten with care. When they are perfectly ripe, bananas are a peerless "dessert" fruit.

I've noticed two things about bananas over the years. First, they are on average twice as large as they were in my youth. Second, you peel it, you'll eat it—often in very big bites, making it disappear in no time. So applying the 50 Percent Solution, I cut the banana in half before peeling it, then wrap the exposed end of one half in plastic. I set that aside for another time, perhaps for breakfast the next day or a later dessert. With a bit of practice, half a twenty-first-century banana makes a most satisfying dessert, especially when you treat it as you would a piece of cake or pie. I don't eat it with my fingers. I peel it and set it out on a plate and eat it with a knife and fork. I savor each bite, and I put down my fork between bites. Eating slowly enlarges the experience, alerting my brain to the banana consumption in process. (Hint: A sliver of banana tastes just as much like banana as a big chunk. Eat the smallest bite that lets you register taste. Then have another.) Lots of people I know would make that half banana vanish in twenty seconds, but how much satisfaction are they getting? I'd bet I derive more by consuming my half mindfully over the course of a few minutes. Try it.

The principle works with liquid nutrition as well. As I'll describe later at greater length, wine is food, but a food whose great benefits can be negated by immoderate consumption— too much of a good thing. Wine is also my business, an indispensable part of my life and lifestyle. And as everyone knows, French women enjoy it without getting fat. Red wines are rich in the flavonoid called resveratrol, a superpotent antioxidant also found in blueberries. But actually all wines are good for you, and one of the most complex, Champagne, has a few distinctive trace elements and uniquely salubrious effects.

But how much is good for you? Doctors, French and otherwise, suggest having a glass or two (four to eight ounces a day), depending on your size—but having it with food, *bien sûr*. Open a typical 750-milliliter bottle, however, and voilà, you are looking at six glasses. What to do? When we are at home, Edward and I rigorously apply the 50 Percent Solution, because we know that after that first or second glass, it can be deliciously simple to pour a third or more, after which the health benefit is shot. (Okay, the *occasional* third glass won't kill you, but it's still not part of a healthy lifestyle.) So here's how it works.

We started out buying some half bottles (375 milliliters) and kept the empties. Now when we open a new bottle of wine for dinner, the first thing we do is pour half the contents into an empty half bottle and cork it immediately. The wine has seen air for perhaps fifteen seconds. Recapped and usually refrigerated, it will last in top form for days, weeks, and even months.

So we always have one or several capped half bottles on hand for future meals. At dinner, a half bottle is good for about three or perhaps four glasses, total. But remember, wine should be sipped and tasted. A wineglass should never be more than half to two-thirds full: to taste it properly, you need room to swirl it, expose it to the air to soften it, and you want the empty part of the glass trapping the bouquet. Enter the 50 Percent Solution yet again: we drink a half glass at a time, each of us perhaps enjoying two refills from the half bottle. (It is amazing how easy it is to fool ourselves. Three half-glass pours are far more psychologically fulfilling and pleasurable, without a feeling of restraint, than a glass and a half or a single pour into a very large glass.)

The greatest and most memorable wine I've ever experienced was a rare Burgundy served to me in a two-ounce portion—and I remember it to this day! Over the years Edward and I have been fortunate to acquire some pretty decent bottles, and using the half-bottle trick, we have not been shy about opening them, knowing that each can be savored on more than one occasion.

And here's one more example of using the 50 Percent Solution in managing portions. I suspect we all know someone who "adds coffee to her sugar." I know at least two women who routinely add four packets of sugar to each of the several cups of coffee they have every day. And that's for a normal-sized cup. We all need our stimulants, but there are so many better ones than sugar.

With a sweet tooth like mine, I am lucky to have learned from Dr. Miracle to take my coffee without sugar. Order coffee or tea in America, however, and you automatically get a sugar bowl with it. So let the sugar in your coffee lead me to another subject deserving more attention than I gave it in *French Women Don't Get Fat.*

THE INCIDENTAL SWEETNESS OF AMERICAN LIFE

This marvelous anthropological expression I owe to Adam Gopnik, who uses it in his book *Through the Children's Gate,* the story of his family's move back home to New York after years of living in Paris. Everybody, and especially the kids, found so many things in America too sweet. It's true, the French have a much lower tolerance for sweetness than most other peoples. Like saltiness, bitterness, sourness, and what some taste physiologists describe as *umami* (savoriness), sweetness is a broad taste sensation that obscures more particular and subtler tastes (and we French try to be all about the subtlety).

Dessert in France is much likelier to be cheese or fruit than pastry (saving room for a final chocolate square or some bite-sized cookies and the like, called petits fours), the point being to clear the palate—or the table, if we follow the derivation from the Old French, *desservir.* At any rate, the idea never was to drown the taste buds in sweetness and fat. Actually, before the nineteenth century, when sugar became cheap and widely available, truly sweet desserts as most Americans now recognize them would have been strictly for the rich or else a special occasion or holiday treat, not an everyday thing.

Unfortunately, America's problem (and to be fair, it's not just America's problem) of incidental sweetness is not limited to sweets, or even sugar. High-fructose corn syrup makes its way into everything from soft drinks to tomato sauces to supermarket yogurt to fast-food french fries, offering calories but not instant energy that most cells in the body can use. (Glucose, not fructose, is what your cells need.) So the energy tends to be stored as you know what. After trans fats, corn syrup is probably the most offensive fattening ingredient in processed foods. And Americans consume on average forty-five pounds of corn syrup a year! (*En passant,* I should say that most fruit juices, high in naturally occurring fructose, are dangerously fattening for the same reason; the body can't easily use the sugar. So my advice is eat, don't drink, your fruit.)

But back to your morning cup of coffee. A teaspoon of sugar once or twice a day is a reasonable indulgence that won't make anyone fat, but lots of people are conditioned to add several to each cup, as well as to having several cups a day—not a good idea in any case. Once our taste—whether for sweetness, fat, salt—is recalibrated over time, an excess that used to taste good comes to taste awful.

Edward always took his coffee with a teaspoon or two. That's how he was raised. One day when he was about to put a heaping teaspoon of sugar into his cup, I asked him if he could drink his coffee without sugar. He looked at me and asked, "Would you eat french fries without ketchup?" (I said, "Yes, I do.") He had never even thought about it. Some days later, I suggested he cut the sugar in half and try it.

He saw it as a challenge. He did, and enjoyed the coffee just the same. Within a few months, he had cut the half in half, and for the past ten or fifteen years he has taken his morning coffee (his only coffee of the day) with no sugar but plenty of pleasure. Deploying the 50 Percent Solution is an effective way to reduce these calories while helping you build up a greater sensitivity to sweetness. (Sugar substitutes, by contrast, while not fattening, only preserve our preternatural taste for the sweet—they are therefore an *un*-useful self-deception.) Eventually you will find the taste of added sugar cloying. You may discover that you actually like the true flavor of coffee.

I have a theory about how we originally came to sweeten our coffee, which the French generally don't do. When I came to America, the coffee was simply awful: poorly made, often from inferior blends, over-roasted beans, stale grounds. It was burned in percolation and reburned in keeping it warm all day. (Freshly brewed coffee holds its peak flavor for about twenty minutes.) So the standard was a bitter pill, strong and caffeine-infused. You needed to add sugar to get it down. Nowadays—thanks to all sorts of beans; better roasting and preservation techniques; and grinders, pods, drip filter coffee-makers, and pressure gadgets; and especially to Starbucks and other such chains—excellent coffee is an affordable luxury. Who would have thought that people would be willing to pay more for quality? I'm sure that idea sounded pretty wacky when first uttered in the elevator.

If you have to travel on business, not even the 50 Percent Solution will help you before the sprawling, unlimited servings of any decent hotel's breakfast buffet. Let me confess: I love it. But I avoid it. I believe in a good breakfast. Without one, you're bound to snack or overeat at lunch.

I've found two safe ways of dealing with the buffet behemoth. First, I make breakfast or brunch at a buffet a special occasion, not a regular occurrence, even when the breakfast comes free. I order room service. It's the same food, and I can eat only what they deliver, which is what I want in the first place.

When I do indulge, I indulge fully but compensate at lunch and perhaps even dinner. (It is all part of thinking about and adjusting food intake over a two- or three-day period. While we should try to balance on a daily basis, that's much harder to do 365 times a year.) I still protect myself from getting carried away by not packing my plate, but instead making a series of trips around the buffet and sitting down between each "course." My advice: Make a first pass without a plate. Fly one reconnaissance mission to see what really looks good, then work out in your head what you're going to have. When I do this, I don't load up in one shot but fly three sorties—say, one for yogurt and fresh berries, another perhaps for oatmeal or for scrambled eggs (or I should say egg, as I usually ask for one egg, never three). After that, I'm usually no longer hungry. But if I do fly a third sortie to "try" the croissant (you never know) or some specialty dish, that's okay. Being perfectly aware of what I'm doing, I just enjoy the buffet and skip the guilt. As a grown-up, I am sure to balance the intake account later that day or the next. Compensations. Not a catastrophe.

On no account would even the most accomplished French woman dream of facing two buffets in one day! Not only is it too disorienting, but those colossal lunch and dinner steam-table affairs just don't have the allure of breakfast. Simply not worth the confrontation. But if you indulge—and we are all invited to functions with buffet meals—remember the three-sortie-rule strategy. Final advice: use only appetizer plates, and treat the offerings as tapas.

LA GYM

The modern hotel suggests another useful parable. A young woman in my office recently said that when she travels for business, "the diet goes out the window." (As with so many familiar expressions, this betrays the sad, unreflective way that "the diet" has become a permanent fixture of life.) But then she said something unexpected: "I always compensate, as you suggest in your book—the hotels have such great fitness centers." She went on to describe how a good hotel often has better machines and classes than her own gym, and so she can't resist the double temptation: eat too much; overdo the exercise, "just to try" every elliptical and Gravitron. There is a fallacy here from the French woman's point of view: exercise is not a compensation for eating; eating is what we do to fuel an active body. Yes, we should all be more active, but "hitting the gym" to offset your calories is backward thinking. It can have the reverse effect of making you a gym addict as well as an overeater.

Gyms are fine if you like that sort of thing (they are somewhat social and give people pleasure and activity), but what the body needs by way of exercise is not all that elaborate. You need to get your heart rate up several times a week for about thirty minutes (a French woman's brisk half-hour walk every day will do this just fine). And particularly after age forty, we should all do some resistance training. Light free weights can be used almost anywhere. Your body, too, can be its own resistance machine: basic push-ups, sit-ups, and lunges are excellent and pretty comprehensive. So is my overall favorite exercise for body and mind, yoga. If you move in order to eat, rather than eat in order to move, you are in effect running yourself into the ground. The French woman's lifestyle is an active one, but it requires that you learn to adjust your intake to support a normal and healthy level of exertion.

This is the meaning of equilibrium, the point at which one can feel *bien dans sa peau.* I may have forgotten to tell you that in the management of their equilibrium French women are especially good at automatically regulating their metabolism. They are most definitely not all naturally endowed with perfectly calibrated ones. With their frequent walks and trips up and down stairs, French women give several boosts to their metabolic rates in the course of each day. Even those many drinks of water require the metabolism to perk up (they don't just make you feel full). So instead of grueling intervals of burning off massive numbers of calories several times a week, French women consume fewer calories and routinely rev the engine higher without even slipping into spandex. In the race of the tortoise and the hare, the French woman is definitely the tortoise.

All women are not created equal, of course. Women are different—unique indeed—coming in all shapes and sizes, and being *bien dans sa peau* is an individual determination and more important than being skinny. Being overweight to the point that it is a short- or long-term danger to your health is not something I condone, of course, but I forget to say often enough that if you are comfortable being *un peu ronde* (a tad overweight) and you are content, so be it. I believe in living and eating more joyfully.

Today, there is some truth to the glib assertion that age fifty is the new forty. (I'm somewhat more dubious about the Beverly Hills nip/tuck-based claim that sixty is the new forty.) There's no denying that women are extending their careers, even their biological clocks, past the point that would have seemed possible even a decade ago. Enjoying the full benefits of these opportunities requires that we pace ourselves, not overdoing our food and drink, our work, or our exercise. But sometimes being fifty is being fifty. I was recently reminded of that last New Year's Eve when I ate and drank like I did when I was thirty-five. I lived to regret it the next day. No matter if in my head I feel like I did ten or twenty years ago, I have to listen to my body sometimes. And I cannot indulge the way I once did without paying a price. A thirty-five-year-old probably feels the same about her twenty-year-old self. Certainly it is okay to indulge or overindulge once in a while, knowing that you are doing so. I didn't. I was not living in my current real world or being *bien dans ma peau.*

Cultivating a positive emotional outlook is vital, too: studies of centenarians find them overwhelmingly to be life-long optimists, in many cases despite having faced crushing adversity. Indeed, cultivation of outlook, as of taste and proportion—of all aspects of the self, really—is the key to *l'art de vivre* (the art of living). French women don't get fat because they know the secret of pleasure. But the secret *to* pleasure is cultivation: a life of ongoing exploration, experimentation, practiced enjoyment, and—most important—self-discovery.

None of us is born appreciating the finer things as fully and satisfyingly as we might. How are we, then, to make our way to the good life? The prescription hasn't changed much in twenty-five hundred years, though French women have kept the faith better than most. *Connais-toi toi-même*—Know Thyself, as the Delphic oracle advised.

The key is also being true to your unique outward self (in addition to your inward emotional self), developing your own style, a look and manner that feels comfortable and right to you and that you are happy to present to the world. You are your own brand. What's your brand's DNA, and how is it expressed? Clothes? Jewelry? Makeup? Hair? Voice? Laugh? Touch? All of the above, and more. I have a good friend who always wears hats—fall, winter, summer, spring. Another woman I know has a collection of lizard brooches and always wears one. As for me: scarves, necklaces, sunglasses—I couldn't be me without them . . . and not being twenty, I no longer dress like a twenty-year-old. (If you do and you are not, you are certainly making a brand statement.) So too is someone who wears lots of makeup or large costume jewelry (or large precious jewelry, for that matter) or carrot-colored hair (which you will see in Paris). Some work, some don't. You have to decide for yourself. For instance, I don't wear jeans. They're just not my style.

No satisfaction is more elemental, more vital to well-being, than the pleasure we seek in what we eat. In *French Women Don't Get Fat,* I provided a thumbnail understanding of the importance of seasonality to the French woman's lifestyle. But as I may have forgotten to tell you, seasonality is far more than knowing what's in season and appreciating nature's best from month to month, important as that is. Seasonality is a manner of being that is responsive to all conditions and stimulations of our environment throughout the year. Learn it, and you will enjoy peak experience. The well-diverted senses have no need of the consolations of excess and inferior experience. Learn and even time will be on your side: a full experience never feels hurried. Eating with pleasure is about pacing yourself during the meal. Losing weight is a matter of finding your equilibrium of intake and exertion week by week. But the plan for life involves us in the perpetual cycle of adjustment that is the seasons of the year. The art of living is pacing yourself in the long run.

How do you keep track of time? Do you measure it out in coffee spoons like Eliot's hapless J. Alfred Prufrock? Is a season to you eight or fifteen new episodes of some reality TV show? For French women, the most elemental cultivation of pleasure traditionally comes from living as mindfully as possible of the annual progression of the natural cycle.

Now, it's true that the four seasons French women observe are not the same all over the world. Much of mankind lives in the tropical zone, where the seasons are reduced to a rainy and a dry time. Even in our temperate zone the seasons can be a variable experience: in most places, winter is the most barren and lifeless; in others, it is relatively mild and summer is the time of greatest hardship. I point this out in recognition of the fact that the seasons as I represent them, and as I experience them living in the United States and France, are not the seasons of every woman's reality—even though people with weight problems are overwhelmingly concentrated in the temperate zone, which comprises most of the developed world. The secret is to master the variations that the year presents where you live, and to live in each interval to the fullest.

There are things in the recitation of my year that I hope you will recognize and wish to adopt, and certainly lots of delicious recipes you can follow practically anywhere. The menus are suggestions, as suitable for losing weight (following the other advice in *French Women Don't Get Fat*) as for maintaining equilibrium. But the larger point is to give you a way of thinking about the way you live, first and foremost in relation to the passage of time. There are seasons of the earth, but also, as Keats pointed out, seasons of the mind, and these exist wherever you may be. Observe them, tune in to them: not only will your satisfactions multiply but they will become fuller, too.

As I've suggested, so many of our woes are rooted in our modern imperative to beat the clock, a fight we feel we've lost before we even begin. As a result, time has no meaning, only cost. The most repeated complaint I heard in connection with *French Women Don't Get Fat* was "Who has the time [to buy and cook food]?" ("I can't find leeks" was a distant second.) What you should come to understand, however, is that time is not something we are given; it is something we make. We all have more to do than can possibly get done in a day. Even French families have been forced to choose which meals they will have *en famille;* the time-honored ritual can no longer be observed with the traditional regularity. The world is no longer set up to furnish such occasions; we make them for ourselves. We must: life would lose all satisfaction without the time we set aside— the days and hours and even the odd moment—that we reserve to enjoy it. This is not selfishness; it is just living, an opportunity too precious to waste.

See whether it doesn't make sense to you as the year progresses.

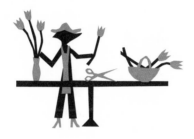

2

When does your year begin? My husband is an academic, and all his life, September has marked the start of the year. So, since our marriage, the end of summer has inevitably marked the start of something for me, too. And some of us never lose the foreboding that accompanies the start of a new school term. French kids are no different, fending off despair at the approach of *la rentrée*—literally, the reentry, as if summer were a trip to the moon.

The corporate world's fiscal years also don't always match the calendar year. For decades my year, at least professionally, has been defined as an annual budget. *C'est normal:* making order from the chaos of our time is quite human as long as we remember that each order we invent serves a particular master.

For thousands of years before electrical power, nature ruled overtly. The days were defined by the appearance and disappearance of the sun, the year by changes in the height of its arc at midday. Springtime, when the days start gaining on the nights, was always the natural start of the year, which explains why in French it's called *printemps,* the first time, and *en italien, primavera.* Today spring is still seen as a time of regeneration, when we wipe the cold sleep from our eyes and awaken to the elaborate interplay of new sensory stimuli: light, fragrances, tastes, sounds. To live according to the season is to be alert to this awakening, not to sleep through it. We can't help responding to the sunlight on our face, but there is infinitely more for the senses to register. Cultivating attention to the full spectrum of sensations affords French women a wealth of slimming experience, of compensations and distractions. Day by day, there is so much to take in, so much potential pleasure, that they become less vulnerable to mindless eating and its consequence, getting fat. That works out pretty well as the forgiving layers of winter are being peeled off.

With the arrival of spring produce in the market comes the prospect of many gastronomic pleasures. But for me, the most precious heralds of spring are flowers. I count the days until the crocuses will pop up their little heads and cherry blossoms will appear seemingly overnight, their petals scattering almost at once to cover the ground like a snowfall. When I observe the dance of the tulips and daffodils, something stirs within me.

I may sound like a Romantic poet, but you should understand: I grew up with flowers, some cultivated in our huge garden, others found in the fields and woods surrounding my grandmother's house in Alsace. Next to cooking, flowers were my mother's great passion; she couldn't live without them. Neither can I, whatever the season. Like meals, they were part of our daily rituals. I loved learning their names, picking them, and helping *Mamie* create her gorgeous, unfussy bouquets. Early on, I was taught the loving care they demand once taken from the garden and placed in a vase. As a little girl I learned to cut the stem diagonally and change the water every other day. And in a big house with flowers in every room, this was no small chore. But to handle them, to smell them as they opened until the bloom was off them, intensified the experience of having them around. It still does.

As fortune would have it, I married someone who enjoys flowers as much as my mother did. On Saturday mornings in springtime, our sensory nourishment includes going to the greenmarket to bring home some of these perfect tokens of the first season. Flowers don't have to be expensive, and you don't need tons: as in all things, less can be more. One or two simple stalks of sweet peas in a small vase can provide great pleasure, adding a dash of color and a delicately sweet scent to a room.

Flowers, *Mamie* told me, are very much like us, none more so than the tulip. Tulips smile at you, talk to you, let you know when they need water, have too much light; and before they die, they are at their most serenely beautiful, stems flagging as if reaching out for a final embrace, the folding petals expressing in their contortions every imaginable emotion. Just look at them. The shapes are fascinating: the small, round petals and the pointed ones; the so-called long-stemmed French tulips and my favorite, the parrot tulip. As for colors, tulips, like roses, come in an astonishing variety, and I can remember every one in our garden. The first spring tulip announced to me what was coming. Tulips still lift my spirits when I see them in a vase, though never more than when I see them rising from the earth in springtime.

By then, I am delirious with spring fever. I find myself buying armfuls of flowers, drinking in scents and colors. The vernal mania extends even to selecting more brightly colored linens for the bed and table, putting away the austere monochromes or crisp whites I love in winter. Fortunately, I have long been in the habit of undertaking spring cleaning in late winter (actually very therapeutic exertion on a gray Saturday afternoon). By springtime, I know where everything is to be found in the closets, and I won't find myself doing chores when all I want is to be outside.

In spring, there is no excuse for not making the most of a French woman's most powerful equilibrium manager: walking. Even during April showers, I love being out and about. And when the weather is clear, the possibilities multiply, and it's time to take out the bike. This past spring, many people who could have sworn they lived in car towns took to their bikes as the price of gasoline soared. (It's a matter not of what's possible but of what's imaginable.)

Cycling has well-known health benefits: it's a low-impact, mild aerobic exercise that strengthens your heart and lungs; tones the large (read: fat-burning) muscle groups; keeps joints, tendons, and ligaments flexible; builds stamina; and is generally fun, reducing stress and boosting your mood. But in northern climes—France included—it's just not a safe or comfortable year-round activity, at least, not for me. I cross off winter, which makes my first ride in spring something to look forward to.

French and other European women are much more likely to use bicycles for conveyance than are Americans, who see cycling more as recreation and sport. Remember, the French invented the Tour de France yet still have not forgotten the practical uses of the bike. For my mother's generation (and those like the 122-year-old Jeanne Louise Calment), riding was something women did every day. When you think of it, most commutes today are under five miles, less than thirty minutes by bike. Cycling is something Edward and I can do together just for fun, but anyone who can do it for more practical reasons should.

We rarely bicycle in New York or Paris anymore, except a bit on weekends, when there's less traffic. But when we were younger, we would pedal regularly through the side streets of Greenwich Village and on the bike path along the Hudson River when heading up- or downtown. Even more regularly, we'd cart the bikes to the country. Nowadays, most of our cycling is done in Provence, where the view, the feel of rolling hills, and the olfactory splendors give us the potent sensation of being beyond workaday cares, outside of ourselves. In fact, I feel that way anytime I am *en vélo*. It requires just enough attention to concentrate the mind pleasantly, and I have never lost the child's thrill at propelling myself faster than my legs could carry me—quite a different pleasure from motoring.

This past winter, Edward surprised me with a new silver-and-black bike from Peugeot, legendary maker of bicycles (not just automobiles) for more than a century. He selected and purchased the bicycle secretly, then gave me a picture of it in

New York on Valentine's Day, with a nice bicycle poem as well; the real thing was delivered to our home in Provence and was there to greet me when I arrived. Though the official start of spring was a few days off, I just could not resist taking the Peugeot for an inaugural spin. There was still a chill in the air, but in the sun I didn't mind at all. I went all the way to the market.

Au marché, where French women observe the arrival of springtime most seriously: nothing is more meaningful than our choice of what to consume as the grip of winter yields.

For centuries French women felt springtime's anticipation even more keenly than they do now. Since the Middle Ages, the predominantly Catholic population observed a Lenten fast. Mardi Gras (Fat Tuesday) was less the bacchanal staged in New Orleans or Rio and more what it was conceived to be: the last day that meat and other foods, including eggs and dairy, could be enjoyed before the forty-day period of abstinence between Ash Wednesday and Easter. Those would-be French women who have balked at the rigors of my Magical Leek Soup weekend might do well to consider the virtues of traditional French ways. During Lent, not only did one forgo the richest foods, but those young enough to endure it took only one daily meal, at the end of the workday. (Charlemagne, by imperial prerogative, took his at 2 p.m.; it's good to be the king!) While I, a latter-day French woman of Huguenot extraction, would hardly prescribe a regimen so severely penitential, it does suggest to me a reason why traditionally French women don't get fat. Like a prolonged version of the Magical Leek weekend, the Lenten fast would reset the body's dials, making it more alert to the tastes it can enjoy and, eventually, more appreciative of those that for a time it had to forgo.

Come the *fêtes de Pâques* (Easter), everything enjoyed in celebration was consumed more mindfully. Meanwhile, probably
not a few excess winter pounds had been shed. (The psychol-
ogy of this cultural and spiritual discipline is very different
from the tedium of dieting, a decidedly modern perversion by
which we try to subtract the meals we've already eaten.) After
the fast, every food of springtime, from the fresh vegetables to
the spring lamb, must have tasted like the first. The body
accustomed to less finds that indeed less is more. In fact, a
body conditioned to enjoy less will naturally find excess
unpleasant.

The market is my own lesson in patience as spring
approaches. The time of pears and apples is all too slowly
winding down; I'm getting a bit bored with citrus fruit and
bananas. And although global agribusiness can today summon
forth the fruits of the hemisphere, enjoying its summer in the
midst of our winter, it's somehow not the same as receiving
what comes into its own locally, in sync with all else that is
changing around me. I find myself longing to switch gears with
my menus and start planning the first brunch outdoors.

The march of seasonal produce that begins in spring,
while not quite the equal of summer's bounty, is more than
enough to whet my appetite for the feast of freshness to come:
The first peas in their pods. The first fiddlehead ferns. The
first bunch of crisp spinach. Honestly, fresh local produce is
nothing like what the transnational conglomerates bring to
your supermarket hub. The local version registers true colors
and oozes with subtle flavors. It is produced by people who
will look you in the eye when they sell it to you. And it is
picked and sold when ripe! Now, we don't live in Eden, and

not everything can be as we would have it. But whatever else you eat, if you make it your business to find some such fresh local produce every week, the rewards of its flavors will make the simplest dish satisfying in a modest portion.

I do recognize that this is easier said than done. A couple of hundred years ago, when virtually everyone was a farmer or lived near one, it was easy to acquire these seasonal blessings. Times change, but together with all the improvements to our lives we have inherited a global obesity epidemic. (It seems a cruel truth that people are growing fatter everywhere they aren't starving.)

However much I manage to enjoy nature's bounty, I cannot ignore the impoverishment relative to my childhood, when my father, a white-collar worker and an avid gardener in his spare time, surrounded us with extensive fruit and vegetable plantings. Come spring, before every meal we would gather ripe fruit and vegetables. After dinner it was a family ritual to walk to the garden and admire nature's work. Not that I remember needing one, but this evening stroll was an anti-stress pill par excellence and never failed to put me in a proper frame of mind for a good night's sleep. The twenty-first-century paradise we have tried to create can't hold a candle to such satisfaction, but if nature is no longer at our door, we must go looking for it.

PETITS POIS À POINT

We grew peas in our garden, and so they were another spring treat by which I was spoiled rotten. I would graze on them raw right from the pod as my father picked them, not an hour before they would be served at table. Steamed or boiled and served with a little butter, they regularly furnished "color" on our dinner plates. Peas, like corn, are vegetables that cry out to be bought at farmstands and eaten fresh. When picked, peas (and corn) are rich with natural sugars, but these immediately begin turning to starch. A perfectly ripe just-picked pea is a special sensation. All others might as well be dancing with diced carrots in a can.

BROWN RICE WITH PEAS

Serves 4

1. Cook the rice according to package directions.

2. Warm the oil in a skillet over medium heat. Add the butter, shallots, and lemon zest, and sauté for 5 minutes.

3. Add the peas, and cook until tender, adding a little water if the shallots start to brown before the peas are tender.

4. Add the cooked rice, season with salt and pepper to taste, and stir to combine. Remove from the heat, and add the parsley.

INGREDIENTS

1 cup uncooked brown rice

1 tablespoon olive oil

1 tablespoon unsalted butter

2 tablespoons minced shallots

Zest of ½ lemon

1 pound fresh peas, shelled

Salt and freshly ground pepper

3 tablespoons minced parsley

SPRING PEAS WITH PEARL ONIONS

Serves 4

1 tablespoon olive oil

½ cup pearl onions

2 cups fresh peas, shelled

1 tablespoon herbes de Provence

Salt and freshly ground pepper

1. Warm the oil in a saucepan over low heat. Add the onions, peas, and herbes de Provence. Cook over low heat for 20 minutes, stirring occasionally.

2. Season with salt and pepper to taste, and serve immediately.

· ·

ASPARAGUS

One can find asparagus all year long, but whether from local farmers in New York City's Union Square Greenmarket or Paris's Raspail market or restaurants with seasonal market menus, there's nothing that tastes like spring asparagus. Somewhere, not far from you, the real thing is to be had, ready to compensate for the effort with flavor that is to the supermarket variety as dairy-fresh whipped cream is to Cool Whip.

I've loved asparagus since childhood. It's no surprise: the agreeable rituals and foods we discover as kids remain reference points throughout life (mothers and fathers, take note). In those days, only white asparagus was available. Grown out of sunlight (limiting photosynthesis) and more delicately flavored than the green variety more common in the States, the white stalks were a Sunday lunch treat. My mother would make a mayonnaise from scratch and blanch the asparagus at the last moment, serving them as an appetizer. We each had four to six stalks to dunk in the mayonnaise with our fingers, sucking and chewing till we reached the inedible fibrous end. At the end of the course we'd dunk our fingers in the *rince-doigts*, a little bowl of water with a slice of lemon (to cut the grease) floating in it. It's the subject of many jokes (mostly apocryphal, no doubt) about confused guests uncertain whether to drink from the bowl. But when your fingers are sticky with asparagus and mayonnaise, it is not hard to figure out what the *rince-doigts* is for.

I discovered green asparagus when I came to New York, and my first experience was actually not a happy one, although color had nothing to do with it. Wanting to show off our West Village digs, we invited Edward's sister and her husband to lunch one Saturday in spring. At the market, I had fetched a few bunches (always make sure they are not droopy or browning and that the flowering ends are shut tight). I had decided to make a one-course brunch, *asparagus quiche sans dough*, whose delicious simplicity many American friends had enjoyed immensely. Eggs and asparagus go splendidly together (in fact, a simple poached egg makes a nice *fausse* hollandaise, when whipping up a mayonnaise seems too ambitious for the boiled-asparagus appetizer), and some bacon cubes provide extra tang and color. But when the large white ceramic dish came out of the oven and we sat down to eat, I saw an uncomfortable look on my sister-in-law's face. She was the first person I'd ever met who hated asparagus. I made her an omelet as Edward, sheepish at not having remembered, poured more wine.

Food aversions and allergies seem much more common in America than in France, where in many years of entertaining

I've suffered relatively few such faux pas. You do get the occasional youngster allergic to (or perhaps just grossed out by) seafood. Still, *à chacun son goût,* and since we are preaching a gospel of tastes, it's only right to honor those of our friends. So if you are serving an all-or-nothing dish, especially using a potential allergen, pay heed. (Believe it or not, a French friend of mine is allergic to garlic! Anything is possible.)

Now that I'm fortunate enough to spend a few days in Paris and Provence each March, I can live on asparagus for a week. (Variety is key to the French woman's gastronomy, but the obsessive enjoyment of a particular food briefly in season is no sin, provided the food is not an offender, full of fat or processed sugar. The good news is that almost all vegetables are fair game for occasional monomania.) Fresh green asparagus can be as delicious as our white variety (though the latter still seems more sophisticated when served in the United States). I simply boil or steam them, adding a piece of salted butter (the famous Guérande is itself a luxury) and a touch of freshly ground pepper to the cooked, drained spears, then serve them with some protein, which becomes secondary as I feast on the asparagus. One blessing of seasonal vegetables is that they allow you to be satisfied with smaller amounts of protein—high-energy, low-fiber food that, regardless of Atkins and South Beach advice, can make you fat if taken too liberally without the perverse restriction of carbohydrates. In fact, try to eat your protein first to slow digestion and promote satiety; if you come to think of it as the "side" and the vegetables as the main dish, you will be cluing into a very common trick by which French women stay slim.

WHITE ASPARAGUS WITH MAYONNAISE, *MAMIE*'S VERSION

Serves 4

1. In a warmed bowl (fill it with boiling water and let stand for a few minutes), whisk together the egg yolk, mustard, and vinegar. Slowly, by droplets, whisk in the oil until at least half has gone in and the mixture has the thickness of heavy cream. Continue whisking in the oil, now in a thin but steady stream, until all of it is incorporated. Season with salt and pepper to taste.

2. Serve the asparagus warm on a plate. Decorate with the sprigs of parsley and add 2 tablespoons of mayonnaise per person. This is finger food: dunk each spear in some mayo and enjoy until you get to the end of the stalk, which is tough and may still have some inedible fibers. When you run out of asparagus, use a *rince-doigts* to clean your fingers.

INGREDIENTS

1 egg yolk at room temperature

1 teaspoon Dijon mustard

1 to 2 teaspoons sherry vinegar

$2/3$ to 1 cup canola oil

Fine sea salt

Freshly ground white pepper

16 to 24 white asparagus stalks, peeled and blanched

Fresh parsley

N.B. MANY OF US ARE INTIMIDATED BY THE PROSPECT OF MAKING MAYONNAISE, BECAUSE WE KNOW THAT IF THE OIL ISN'T ADDED SLOWLY ENOUGH, THE MIXTURE MAY CURDLE. TO CORRECT SUCH A SNAFU, JUST PUT ANOTHER EGG YOLK IN A BOWL, ADD THE FAILED MAYO, AND CONTINUE ADDING THE REST OF THE OIL. WHISK WELL. VOILÀ.

N.B. IT IS ADVISABLE NOT TO SERVE DISHES INCORPORATING UNCOOKED EGGS TO PREGNANT WOMEN, SMALL CHILDREN, SENIORS, AND PEOPLE WITH IMMUNE-SYSTEM DEFICIENCIES.

ASPARAGUS AND CASHEW OMELET

Serves 4

INGREDIENTS

2 ounces unsalted raw
cashews, chopped

6 eggs

2 tablespoons water

4 ounces grated cheese
(Swiss or Parmesan)

1 tablespoon coarsely
chopped parsley

Salt and freshly ground
pepper

1 teaspoon olive oil

1 tablespoon unsalted
butter

8 ounces boiled asparagus
tips (green or white)

1. Roast the cashews for a few minutes in a dry frying pan over medium heat to release the flavor. In a bowl, beat the eggs with the nuts, water, cheese, and parsley. Season with salt and pepper to taste.

2. Warm the same pan over medium heat. Add the oil and butter. When the butter melts, pour in the egg mixture and cook, letting it sit until it is softly set but still moist. Add the asparagus tips and cook 4 to 5 minutes longer. Serve immediately.

. . . .

ASPARAGUS WITH HONEY SAUCE

Serves 4

INGREDIENTS

½ teaspoon salt

1 pound fresh asparagus,
bottom inch cut off

1. Fill a saucepan large enough to hold the asparagus with water. Add the salt and bring the water to a boil. Add the asparagus and cook with the lid on until barely tender, about 3 minutes. Drain.

2. Combine the mustard, honey, shallot, and thyme, and mix well. Pour over the asparagus, and serve.

INGREDIENTS

¼ cup Meaux mustard

2 tablespoons honey

1 tablespoon minced shallot

Pinch of fresh thyme

N.B. MEAUX MUSTARD IS MADE FROM CRUSHED MUSTARD SEEDS RATHER THAN FROM SEEDS GROUND TO A POWDER, AND IT IS GENERALLY MILD. IN CONTRAST, DIJON IS LIGHT IN COLOR AND FAIRLY STRONG IN FLAVOR. I PREFER MEAUX FOR ITS COLOR, TEXTURE, AND TASTE.

. . . .

FETTUCCINE WITH SCALLOPS AND ASPARAGUS

Serves 4

1. Bring 8 cups of salted water to a rolling boil in a large pot. Cook the pasta following package directions. Add the asparagus to the pot during the last minute of cooking. Drain the pasta and asparagus, and set aside.

2. Warm a large skillet over medium heat, and add 1 tablespoon of the oil. Add the scallops, and cook 3 minutes. Turn the scallops, and cook 3 minutes more, or until

INGREDIENTS

10 ounces fettuccine

Salt and freshly ground pepper

16 asparagus stalks, trimmed and sliced diagonally into 2-inch pieces

2 tablespoons olive oil

¾ pound scallops, rinsed and dried on paper towels

INGREDIENTS

Zest and juice of 1 lemon

2 tablespoons basil, chopped

seared. Remove the scallops from the pan, and set aside.

3. In the same skillet over low heat, combine lemon zest and juice and the remaining oil. Add the pasta, asparagus, and scallops, and toss well. Season with salt and pepper to taste. Garnish with basil. Serve immediately.

· ·

MORE PASTA, PLEASE

Pasta, like other carbs, has in the past year or two been rehabilitated. At the same time, food manufacturers (the oxymoron says it all) have rushed to clear the shelves of their low-carb science projects. But that doesn't mean it's totally safe to go back in the water. Individuals who haven't forsworn pasta (and no one should) are still well advised to use their heads. It is, as the nutritionists say, a relatively high glycemic food. (I have scant use for glycemic indexing, much less the GI Diet, whose name alone probably puts me off: a friend had to correct my impression that the initials stand for the Gastro-Intestinal Diet.) Suffice it to say, pasta does elevate the insulin level and so *can* produce cravings for more and more. Loving it so much, I count it as one of my offenders, something I'm prone to overdo without proper care. Especially in a post-low-carb world, it's important not to lapse into carb abuse.

When I was growing up, we had pasta a few times a month. Since children naturally love it, my mother saw it as a way to make us eat our vegetables. Being a working woman, she developed a few one-dish meals for hectic days (eating in courses is optimal, but in a pinch you can achieve a balanced variety of satisfying foods in one dish). We would get carbohydrates (though no bread was on the table when pasta was served), a leftover piece of chicken or tuna or calf's liver was chopped in to take care of our protein needs, and the all-important vegetables were let in the back door. In terms of flavor they were the true stars of the dish, though all we knew was that we were eating *pasta.*

Still, I don't think it was until I started traveling to Italy with my husband that I truly fell in love with pasta. One summer, while Edward was working on a photo exhibition at Casa Guidi, the Browning home in Florence, we lived in a small hotel along the Arno, in a big room with a view from the terrace. And what a view it was: just above roof level the whole city center spread before our eyes, with the majestic Duomo full-frame and the surrounding hills beyond. *"O bella libertà, O bella!"* as Elizabeth Barrett Browning wrote. Since I wasn't there to work, I was left in charge of meals and entertainment. I quickly discovered that all the small local food shops had marvelous pasta dishes that I could buy just before Edward "came home" for lunch. Every day we had a different pasta, but remembering my mother's example, I'd make sure we also had some greens (for extra vitamins and fiber) and some salami or other protein (to promote satiety). To this day, I can't recall any more elementally perfect meals than those Florentine affairs. Sitting on our little shaded terrace at midday, when everyone in Italy went home for lunch, we enjoyed the most quietly romantic idyll, outside time and worldly cares: warm breezes, good, simple food, a glass of Chianti, and some fruit before settling down for a siesta. Could there be any purer bliss?

Remarkably, we ate pasta every day (sometimes twice a day!), but always in the portion the Italians enjoy, about four ounces. You can easily implement portion control with pasta at home if you weigh it first; no one boils another pot just to eat more pasta, and by the time the water was boiling, you wouldn't be hungry anyway. I advise saving a bit of the cooking water to add later to moisten the pasta and dilute overly rich sauces.

After a month of this we had not gained an ounce. Sure, we were young, and we walked a lot. But all around us were Italians of every age who were eating likewise and generally not overweight. (If only it were still true today, some two or more decades later, but Italy, like France, is headed away from, not toward, the benefits of gastronomic tradition and moderation.) Why didn't the Italians of our youth seem to be fat? Simple: it was all a matter of proportion. Like us, they were having pasta with their other food, not other food with their pasta. The key was to eat not just pasta with some bland marinara and pre-grated Parmesan. These were well-considered, balanced meals, almost sufficient unto themselves, to which pasta had been *added* as a kind of matrix for other things, comprising a wide variety of nutrients and flavors. Eating a relatively small portion of such a "thoughtful" pasta was filling enough to stave off afternoon hunger pangs and snacking: our stomachs, having been taken good care of, were usually content to skip the afternoon gelato treat. When we did have one, we certainly relished it, but never on account of feeling unsatisfied by lunch.

My mother's trick of mixing vegetables with starch is one French women still deploy, especially as a vegetable delivery system for children. Brillat-Savarin said, *"Le nombre des saveurs est infini"* (there is an infinite number of flavors). So it is with vegetables and pasta: there is no limit to the ways they can be blended. The vegetables bring the fiber (soluble for slowly released energy, insoluble for bulk and satiety), and the pasta brings a quicker complex-carb energy fix; together they are the perfect time-release package. Ask any endurance athlete.

Recently Edward and I went to dinner at a good neighborhood Italian restaurant in the seventh arrondissement near the Eiffel Tower. It is owned and run by two sisters from Bergamo, helped by an elderly Chinese waiter. The clientele was strictly French, and the place was so packed it was turning away drop-ins—not so common at French restaurants without Michelin stars. Two local couples who had reserved came in with their children, four in all, between the ages of six and twelve, I'd say. The kids had a pasta course, then left. "Call me on my cell as soon as you get home," the father, still enjoying his appetizer, said to the eldest. Although the kids' dine-and-dash wasn't my idea of a meal properly enjoyed *en famille,* I couldn't help noting that the pasta had proved itself once again as a fail-safe way to feed the young. And I heard myself, perhaps the kid in me, say, "You know, Edward"—actually, in France I call him Édouard—"I could eat pasta every day." I really could, but I don't. I was enjoying a first course of spaghetti with langoustines. Edward had spaghetti carbonara. We tried each other's dish, and both were excellent. Fortunately, my inner French woman and not my inner child still calls the shots—usually. I content myself with pasta once every week or so.

SPAGHETTI WITH FIDDLEHEAD FERNS AND PROSCIUTTO

Serves 4

Fiddlehead ferns are a spring delicacy you probably won't find in your supermarket. The ostrich fern and a few other varieties are edible and in spring send out shoots that are tightly curled at their ends before the leaves unfurl. They look like the scroll of a lute or fiddle. Where there are woods, there are ferns, and if you live in driving distance of woodland, chances are your specialty grocer or farmers' market will carry them. But don't blink or you'll miss them: the season is short, and they are highly perishable. At New York's Union Square Greenmarket, where I first encountered them, I also learned that they were something of a New England delicacy, since pre-Colonial times a staple in the local Native American diet. They are also eaten traditionally in Asia, Australia, and New Zealand. They are decidedly not French, however, and have the look of something that defies you to divine a way to prepare them. Fortunately, the farmer with his basket of fiddleheads at Union Square was forthcoming and saved me the trial and error. Once I mastered them— very simple to do, actually—it took only a short French woman's leap to try them with pasta. Now they are something we look forward to, if ever so briefly, in spring.

1. Cook the spaghetti according to package directions. Drain and set aside, reserving ½ cup of cooking water.

2. Add the reserved water to the skillet with the cooked fiddleheads, and mix well. Add the prosciutto, and cook 2 minutes more while stirring.

3. Toss the pasta with the fiddlehead sauce, transfer to a serving bowl, sprinkle with Parmesan and parsley, season with salt and pepper to taste, and serve immediately.

INGREDIENTS

16 ounces spaghetti

Fiddlehead Ferns (recipe follows)

2 ounces prosciutto or pancetta, cut into small pieces

4 tablespoons grated Parmesan

2 tablespoons chopped parsley

Salt and freshly ground pepper

N. B. IF YOU CAN'T FIND FIDDLEHEAD FERNS, BROCCOLI RABE IS AN ALTERNATIVE.

FIDDLEHEAD FERNS

Serves 4

INGREDIENTS

2 cups fiddlehead ferns
2 tablespoons olive oil
2 cloves garlic, minced
1 tablespoon lemon juice
Salt and freshly ground
pepper

1. Clean the fiddleheads thoroughly by washing them several times in cold water to get rid of the brown coat some of them have. Steam them for 6 minutes.

2. Warm the oil in a skillet over medium-high heat. Add the garlic, fiddleheads, and lemon juice. Season with salt and pepper to taste, and sauté, stirring, for 5 to 10 minutes, until the fiddleheads absorb the flavors of the garlic and lemon. Be careful not to overcook. Serve as an accompaniment to meat dishes or as part of the preceding pasta dish.

. . . .

PAPPARDELLE WITH SPRING VEGETABLES

Serves 4

Whenever I make this, I am reminded of pasta primavera (spring pasta), a dish that became all the rage in America in the 1980s and remains to this day something of a classic. The genesis (at least for the name) can be traced to our friends Sirio and Egi Maccioni, owners of the legendary Le Cirque restaurant in New York. The story goes like this: In the late 1970s, Sirio and Egi and some friends, including Pierre Franey and Craig Claiborne, then both food writers at the New York Times, *found themselves in Canada in a house with not much to eat (that's a story in itself). Luckily, Egi and Pierre, true culinary magicians, were wonders at concocting meals from practically nothing. They found pasta and a can of peas and some fresh vegetables and . . . well, the rest is history. It's actually not such an unusual story. As with so many now standard dishes, necessity was the mother of invention. The only difference is that Sirio—running what was then one of the most famous restaurants in the world, a cafeteria for ladies who lunch as well as titans of industry and government—had a bit more influence than the proprietor of the average mom-and-pop eatery. Though Tuscan by birth, he was famed for his impeccable temple of French haute cuisine, and so it was nothing less than* scandale *when he decided to add his impromptu farmhouse pasta to its menu. His French chef refused to make it. (I believe he may have humored Sirio by producing various versions that turned out to be completely* dégueulasses—*ridiculously horrible.) But Sirio eventually gets what he wants, and being a great showman, he came up with the idea of preparing the dish tableside. So take* zat, *you French chef. The pasta primavera was never on the menu, though it was occasionally announced as a special and always available on demand. If you are a tastemaker like Sirio and you feature something new, the speed of the knockoffs, as in the fashion business, could make your head spin. Eventually pasta primavera reached not only the West Coast but the Old World as well, remaining a standard in both hemispheres, though there is no classic recipe, except pasta and spring vegetables. Unbeknownst to him, Sirio was adventurously channeling the adaptive spirit of French women without borders. Sirio's original was made with spaghetti, a cream sauce, and chopped tomatoes; my variation is but an homage.*

1. Blanch the asparagus in salted water until just tender, about 5 minutes. Blanch the peas separately for about 1 minute.

INGREDIENTS

1 pound green asparagus (bottom inch cut off), sliced in half crosswise

2 cups fresh peas, shelled

INGREDIENTS

2 tablespoons minced shallots

¼ cup extra-virgin olive oil

12 ounces (4 cups) pappardelle

¼ cup toasted pine nuts

½ cup freshly grated Parmesan

¼ cup roughly chopped parsley

Coarse sea salt and freshly ground pepper

2. In a heavy saucepan, gently sauté the shallots in the oil over medium-low heat until they begin to turn golden. Add the peas and asparagus, and cook for a few minutes.

3. Cook the pappardelle according to package directions, drain, and toss in the saucepan with the vegetables. Add the pine nuts, Parmesan, and parsley, and season with salt and pepper to taste. Serve immediately.

. . . .

"AY, LEEKS IS GOOD"

Leeks: the star vegetable of *French Women Don't Get Fat,* whose publication actually caused many a local run on them—no joke. You would think the French owned the rights to the leek, which enjoys almost noble rank in France. *Le poireau* is both the vegetable and what they call the green-and-white ribbon of the Ordre national du mérite agricole, the national honor for distinction in food, wine, or agriculture. But the leek is also the staple and historical symbol of the Welsh (see Prince Charles's escutcheon) and makes a memorable appearance in *Henry V* (act 5, scene 1), when King Harry's faithful Fluellen defends his Welsh pride using the vegetable as a cudgel and delivers himself of the ungrammatical truism "Ay, leeks is good." A few more words are due this most distinguished bulb, with its slightly sweet, oniony, even nutty taste, its wealth of nutrients, and its mildly diuretic effect (a secret I have been doing my best to expose).

In France we consume leeks most of the year, except from August to October. In winter they are huge, and we avoid the fattest ones as they are often too fibrous. In spring and summer they tend to be thin and tender and are followed by the *poireaux baguettes,* a very skinny variety. Come spring, ah, the farmers' markets abound with them—lately the baby leeks called ramps have been the season's first celebrity sightings.

The local leek shortages in America that followed the introduction of my Magical Leek Soup were truly *incroyables,* especially when one commentator predicted speculation on the commodities exchange. But when several health magazines published the recipe with a photo of whole leeks cooking in a pot, I knew there was still work to be done in bringing the leek stateside. When cooking with this mild and refined form of garlic, you should cut away and discard the green: the white bulb and the white part of the stalks are the edible part! With that off my chest, let me add that a world of possibilities is open to you with leeks, the Magical Leek Soup from *French Women Don't Get Fat* being only the most Spartan alternative (though still a good one for recapturing your equilibrium from time to time, as we all need to).

MAGICAL LEEK SOUP (BROTH)

Serves 1 for the weekend

INGREDIENTS

2 pounds leeks

1. Clean the leeks and rinse well to get rid of sand and soil. Cut off the ends of the dark green parts, leaving all the white parts plus a suggestion of pale green. (Reserve the extra greens for soup stock.)

2. Put the leeks in a large pot and cover with water. Bring to a boil, reduce the heat, and simmer, uncovered, for 20 to 30 minutes. Pour off the liquid and reserve. Place the leeks in a bowl.

N.B. THIS IS A DETOX WEEKEND, NOT TO BE OVERDONE. DON'T BE TEMPTED TO DO IT OVER AND OVER. I RECOMMEND ONCE A QUARTER.

IF YOU ARE USED TO A HIGH-CALORIE INTAKE EACH DAY, YOU MAY OBVIOUSLY FEEL HUNGRY AND TIRED. SO NO JOGGING OR STRENUOUS ACTIVITIES. RESTING, READING, AND RELISHING IS WHAT THIS WEEKEND IS ABOUT.

FOR THOSE WHO CAN'T LIVE ON LEEK SOUP FOR THE WHOLE WEEKEND, ONE DAY EVERY TWO MONTHS IS GOOD, ALTHOUGH IT WON'T HAVE QUITE THE SAME EFFECT. A TYPICAL FRENCH WOMAN WILL DO THE LEEK WEEKEND TWO TO FOUR TIMES A YEAR.

. . . .

The juice is to be drunk (reheated or at room temperature to taste) every 2 to 3 hours, 1 cup at a time.

For meals, or whenever hungry, have some of the leeks themselves, ½ cup at a time. Drizzle with a few drops of extra-virgin olive oil and lemon juice. Season sparingly with salt and pepper. Sprinkle with chopped parsley if you wish.

This will be your nourishment for both days, until Sunday dinner, when you can have a small piece of meat or fish (4 to 6 ounces—don't lose that scale yet!), with 2 vegetables, steamed with a bit of butter or olive oil, and a piece of fruit.

Leeks are so versatile, I guarantee you'll find your own uses once you get to know them. Meanwhile, a few more of my favorite recipes follow.

OYSTERS ON STEAMED LEEKS

Serves 4

1. Preheat the oven to 300 degrees.

2. Clean the leeks, and slice thinly. Steam for 4 minutes and set aside.

3. Scrub the oyster shells and discard any that remain open. Spread closed oysters on a baking sheet over a layer of salt (to hold them in place). Put the sheet in the preheated oven for a few minutes, until the oysters open. Remove the meat from the shells, and reserve and strain the liquid. Preheat the broiler.

4. Nestle the steamed leeks into half of the shells, top with oysters, then cover with the remaining half shells and set aside.

5. Prepare the sauce by cooking the oyster juice with the wine until reduced by half.

INGREDIENTS

½ pound leeks, white parts only

24 oysters

4 ounces white wine

INGREDIENTS

2 egg yolks

8 tablespoons unsalted butter

Salt and freshly ground pepper

Off the heat, add the egg yolks, then whisk in the butter to obtain an unctuous consistency. Season with salt and pepper to taste.

6. Put the closed oysters under the broiler for 30 seconds. Remove the top shells, and top each full bottom shell with a tablespoon of sauce. Serve immediately with a warm baguette and the rest of the bottle of wine.

. . . .

LEEKS FETTUCCINE

Serves 4

INGREDIENTS

3/4 pound fettuccine

6 tablespoons olive oil

1 pound leeks, white parts only, sliced into 1-inch pieces

4 ounces Parmesan cheese, freshly grated

Salt and freshly ground pepper

8 thin slices of prosciutto

1. Cook the fettuccine in salted water according to package directions.

2. Meanwhile, warm the oil in a skillet. Sauté the leeks over medium-high heat until translucent.

3. When the pasta is ready, toss it with the leeks, add the cheese, and season with salt and pepper to taste. Serve immediately with the prosciutto as a garnish.

. . . .

LEEK AND SPINACH "QUICHE"

Serves 4

1. Preheat the oven to 350 degrees.

2. Discard the outer leaves of the cabbage, and blanch the inner leaves until tender, about 10 minutes (the water need not be salted). Put the cooked leaves on paper towels to cool and dry out, then line a nonstick oven-safe frying pan with the leaves.

3. Sauté the leeks and onions in the oil over medium heat until tender. Add the spinach. Season with salt and pepper to taste. Continue to cook until the spinach has begun to wilt, then drain the vegetables in a colander.

4. Blend the eggs, cream, cheese, and nutmeg, season with salt and pepper to taste, and fold the mixture with the drained vegetables. Carefully pour it into the cabbage-lined pan.

5. Bake in the preheated oven for 25 to 30 minutes or until the quiche is firm to the touch. Allow it to rest for 10 minutes before serving.

INGREDIENTS

1 head savoy cabbage

2 leeks, white parts only, sliced

2 medium onions, peeled and diced

1 tablespoon olive oil

5 ounces spinach, washed and chopped

Salt and freshly ground pepper

2 large eggs

1 cup cream (more may be needed)

1 cup grated Gruyère cheese

Pinch of nutmeg

SHRIMP AND LEEK "MIMOSA"

Serves 4

INGREDIENTS

8 leeks

2 eggs

1 shallot

1 teaspoon Meaux mustard

2 tablespoons red wine vinegar

Pinch of curry

Salt and freshly ground pepper

3 tablespoons olive oil

½ pound shrimp, peeled, deveined, and cooked

1. Clean the leeks thoroughly. Trim them, keeping about 2 inches of the green part in addition to the whites, and boil them in salted water for 6 to 10 minutes, until they are cooked but still firm. Drain and set aside.

2. Cook the eggs for 8 minutes in boiling water, then peel, chop, and set aside.

3. Peel and chop the shallot, and place it in a bowl with the mustard, vinegar, curry, and salt and pepper to taste. Whisk together, then whisk in the oil to make the sauce.

4. Place the shrimp in the center of a serving dish, surrounded by the leeks. Pour the sauce over all, then sprinkle with chopped eggs.

N.B. THIS DISH IS BEST WHEN SERVED WITH LEEKS THAT ARE LUKEWARM. ANOTHER VERSION CALLS FOR CRABMEAT INSTEAD OF SHRIMP, AND IN PROVENCE WE DO THIS RECIPE WITH MARINATED ANCHOVIES. ALL THREE INGREDIENTS MARRY REALLY WELL WITH LEEKS. THE CRABMEAT OFFERS THE MORE ELEGANT DISH, THE ANCHOVIES THE STRONGER AND MORE RUSTIC.

SEA SCALLOPS AND LEEKS
IN CHAMPAGNE SAUCE

Serves 4

INGREDIENTS

4 leeks, white parts only

1 tablespoon unsalted butter

1 tablespoon minced shallot

⅔ cup brut Champagne

Salt and freshly ground pepper

1 tablespoon olive oil

16 sea scallops, rinsed and dried on paper towels

1 tablespoon chopped parsley

1. Clean the leeks thoroughly, then slice them thinly into a chiffonade.

2. Melt the butter in a large pan. Add the shallot, and cook over medium heat for 5 minutes. Add the leeks and Champagne, season with salt and pepper to taste, and let "sweat" 10 to 15 minutes, until the leeks are tender.

3. In a separate pan, warm the oil over medium-high heat. Reduce heat to medium, and sear the scallops 1 minute on each side. Be sure not to overcook the scallops (if you do they'll taste like rubber). Season with salt to taste.

4. Spread the leeks on a serving dish, and top with the scallops. Drizzle with the Champagne sauce, sprinkle with parsley, and serve immediately.

N.B. SERVE THE REMAINING CHAMPAGNE (OR DRY WHITE WINE) AS AN ACCOMPANYING BEVERAGE. ANOTHER OPTION IS TO REPLACE THE PARSLEY WITH SALMON ROE OR–IF YOU WANT TO SPLURGE FOR A SPECIAL OCCASION–CAVIAR, ABOUT 1/2 TEASPOON ON EACH SCALLOP.

LEEKS MOZZARELLA

Serves 4

INGREDIENTS

2 pounds leeks, white parts only

1 cup fresh basil leaves

8 ounces mozzarella

1 to 2 tablespoons olive oil

1 teaspoon wine or sherry vinegar

Salt (preferably freshly ground—fleur de sel works magic) and freshly ground pepper

1. Preheat the broiler.

2. Clean the leeks thoroughly, and boil in salted water 6 to 10 minutes, until cooked but still firm, then drain.

3. Put the leeks in a baking dish, and cover with a layer of basil leaves. Cut the mozzarella into ¼-inch slices, and place atop the basil layer. Put the dish under the preheated broiler, and watch carefully. In 3 to 5 minutes the cheese should start to melt and brown; at this point, remove the dish.

4. Mix the oil and vinegar and drizzle over the mozzarella. Season with salt and pepper to taste. Serve immediately with a slice of country bread.

. . . .

SARDINES WITH CARROTS AND LEEKS

Serves 4

There can scarcely be a health-conscious eater out there who hasn't heard about the benefits of omega-3 fatty acids in fish such as salmon, mackerel, and sardines. Though I'm no doctor, many have asked me about the health benefits of these versus all the dangers one is also told lurk in fish. Here I'm guided by the French woman's principle of everything in moderation: have it once a week. Still, salmon can be pricey, especially if it's wild, which is really the only kind worth eating: some studies indicate that farmed salmon can have eight times the concentrations of environmental toxins as the wild, and only a fraction of the good fats. Yet, as I don't expect the seas to get any cleaner, I fear for what may happen to wild salmon in a generation. For this reason I'm very keen on sardines as a much more affordable alternative. I enjoy the flavor; they're just as rich in omega-3's as wild salmon; and since they're small, they're further down on the food chain, with that much less opportunity to harbor toxins in the creatures they eat. In this dish the accompaniment is simply carrots and leeks, two vegetables found in my fridge most of the year, either cooked or waiting to be. Leftovers are great served on a piece of country bread covered with a slice of Swiss or Cheddar cheese and grilled till the cheese melts.

1. Preheat the oven to 350 degrees.

2. Warm 2 tablespoons of the oil in a large skillet. Add the carrots, and cook over medium heat for 5 minutes. Add ⅓ cup

INGREDIENTS

3 tablespoons olive oil

6 ounces carrots, peeled and thinly sliced

INGREDIENTS

Salt and freshly ground
pepper

10 ounces leeks, white parts
only, thinly sliced

2 tablespoons minced
shallots

1 tablespoon unsalted
butter

12 medium sardines (about
1½ pounds)

1 tablespoon minced fresh
oregano

Juice of 1 lemon

water, season with salt and pepper to taste, and stir in the leeks and shallots. Cover and cook for 5 to 7 minutes, stirring occasionally, until the vegetables are tender. Add the butter, and cook a minute or two more.

3. Put the sardines in one layer in a shallow 9 × 13 baking dish. Drizzle the remaining oil over them, season with salt and pepper to taste, and sprinkle with oregano. Bake 5 to 7 minutes on each side. Drizzle with the lemon juice, and serve with carrots and leeks.

MACKEREL WITH CARROTS AND LEEKS

Serves 4

Mackerel, another salmon alternative, offers fine taste and excellent value. It reminds me of fresh tuna twenty years ago, when it was relatively cheap because few wanted it—before the sashimi-sushi craze, when tuna became "toro" and the price went through the roof, leaving only lesser cuts for those of us not wielding a sushi knife. A mackerel mania may not be far off, so get with it while the getting is still good. The best fishing begins in May or June, and the season runs into fall. (Ditto for sardines.) A lovely Spanish lady who works at a Union Square Greenmarket fish booth gave me the following very simple preparation for this delicious, under-appreciated fish.

1. Make a marinade by combining 2 tablespoons of the oil with the rosemary, shallots, and lemon juice. Pour over the mackerel, and marinate 10 to 20 minutes.

2. Warm the remaining oil in a large skillet, and cook the mackerel over medium heat, about 3 minutes on each side.

3. Season with salt and pepper to taste (be careful not to oversalt, as mackerel is already salty), and serve with the carrot-leek mixture.

INGREDIENTS

3 tablespoons olive oil

4 tablespoons minced fresh rosemary

2 tablespoons minced shallots

Juice of 1 lemon

1½ pounds mackerel fillets

Salt and freshly ground pepper

Carrot-leek mixture from previous recipe

SALMON WITH FENNEL *EN PAPILLOTE*

Serves 4

3 ounces fresh ginger, peeled and cut into thin sticks

Zest and juice of 1 lemon

4 tablespoons olive oil

Salt and freshly ground pepper

2 fennel bulbs, cleaned and sliced thinly

4 salmon steaks, 4 to 5 ounces each

1. Preheat the oven to 400 degrees.

2. Place the ginger, lemon zest and juice, oil, and salt and pepper to taste in a bowl, and mix well.

3. Cut 8 pieces of parchment paper (or aluminum foil) into squares large enough to cover each salmon steak and leave a 2-inch border all around. Put some fennel and a salmon steak in the center of a square and drizzle over with the ginger-lemon mixture.

4. Place the remaining parchment squares on top of the salmon and fold up the edges to form packets. Simply double folding each of the four sides is enough to seal each packet.

5. Put the *papillotes* on a baking sheet, and bake in the preheated oven for 12 to 15 minutes. Set each *papillote* on a plate, and serve.

. . . .

ROAST CHICKEN WITH ENDIVES

Serves 4

1. Preheat the oven to 400 degrees.

2. Season the chicken well inside and out with salt and pepper. Put the lemon rind in the cavity. Drizzle the chicken with the oil, and put it in the preheated oven. Turn twice over the next 30 minutes. Reduce the temperature to 350 degrees, then cook for 20 minutes more. Add the onion and shallots to the pan, cook for 10 minutes, then add the wine. Reduce the temperature to 300 degrees, and cook for 15 minutes more (a total cooking time of 1 hour and 15 minutes).

3. While the chicken cooks, halve the endives lengthwise, brush with 2 tablespoons of melted butter, and place on the broiler. Once they are slightly browned, turn to brown the other side. Remove the endive halves to an oven-safe dish, season with salt and pepper, and add the lemon juice. Put the endives in the oven for 5 minutes, until their hearts are tender.

4. Remove the chicken from the oven, and reserve its juices (you should have about a cup). Carve the chicken, and arrange on a platter with the endives.

5. Add the cooking juice from the endives to

INGREDIENTS

1 3- to 3½-pound chicken

Salt and freshly ground pepper

Rind and juice of 1 lemon

1 tablespoon olive oil

1 red onion, peeled and sliced

2 tablespoons minced shallots

1 cup red wine

6 endives

4 tablespoons unsalted butter, melted

2 tablespoons red wine vinegar

that of the chicken, and strain into a small bowl. Add the vinegar, stir in the remaining butter, and pour over the chicken. Serve immediately.

. . . .

SALADS AND SIDES

DANDELION SALAD

Serves 4

One of the more startling cultural divides between Americans and the French (and Italians, for that matter) remains their respective views on the dandelion. Americans regard the plants mostly as pests; they want only to kill them. The French, however, prefer to eat them. I can recall dandelion traumas in Weston, Massachusetts, where, readers may remember, I first got fat as an exchange student; and years later in Dix Hills, New York, where Edward grew up. Both communities have well-manicured lawns and gardens. The sight of a dandelion on a lawn is met like the eruption of a pimple on a teenage girl's nose: bring on the chemical warfare, consult the experts, kill, kill, kill before it spreads. Dandelions may do nothing for the beauty of Kentucky bluegrass, but their greens are tasty things. Fortunately, there are signs that the gourmands are gaining on the lawn doctors. More and more it is possible for a little French girl in New York, or anyone else, to buy a bag of wild dandelions (or pick some along roadsides or unkempt lawns!). What a treat you have in store, whether enjoying them raw in a salad or sautéed with a bit of olive oil and lemon, as they are served in Greece.

1. Whisk together the shallot, mustard, vinegar, and anchovy. Season with salt and pepper to taste, and whisk in the oil in a slow stream.

2. Toss the dandelion greens with the dressing, and top with Parmesan shavings (you can shave the cheese with a vegetable peeler).

INGREDIENTS

1 teaspoon minced shallot

1 teaspoon Meaux mustard

1 tablespoon red wine vinegar

1 anchovy fillet, minced

Salt and freshly ground pepper

3 tablespoons olive oil

1 bunch of dandelion greens (about 10 ounces), rinsed and dried

1-ounce piece of Parmesan cheese

SALMON-AND-SPINACH SALAD

Serves 4

Where fresh wild salmon is not available, canned sockeye is a suitable alternative to farmed—the French are far from believing everything in a tin is wicked.

INGREDIENTS

1 shallot, minced
Pinch of sea salt
½ cup sherry vinegar
¾ pound uncooked salmon fillets (or smoked salmon or canned salmon)
1 teaspoon Meaux mustard
Freshly ground pepper
2 tablespoons red wine or raspberry vinegar
¼ cup olive oil
¾ pound spinach, washed and dried

1. Mix together the shallot, salt, and sherry vinegar. Pour onto the salmon, and let marinate for at least 1 hour, preferably 3.

2. Drain off the marinade, and cut the salmon into very thin slices. (This step can be done in advance.)

3. For the dressing, mix the mustard and pepper in a bowl with the red wine vinegar. Add the oil, whisking well.

4. Pour the dressing over the spinach in a large bowl, tossing gently. Place the salmon slices all around. Serve with buttered whole wheat toast.

HARICOTS VERTS WITH TOMATOES

Serves 4

1. Warm the oil in a frying pan over medium heat. Add the anchovies and shallots, and cook for 2 minutes. Add the tomatoes, and cook a few minutes more. Season with salt and pepper to taste, then add the basil.

2. Put the steamed haricots verts in a serving dish, and top with the tomato-anchovy mixture. Serve immediately.

INGREDIENTS

2 tablespoons olive oil

4 anchovies, minced

2 shallots, minced

2 medium-sized tomatoes, coarsely sliced

Salt and freshly ground pepper

1 tablespoon minced fresh basil

1 pound haricots verts, steamed for 8 minutes

. . . .

STEAMED ZUCCHINI WITH BASIL

Serves 4

1. Steam the zucchini for 6 minutes.

2. Combine the lemon juice and oil. Season with salt and pepper and whisk well.

3. Place the steamed zucchini in a serving dish, and top with the dressing and Parmesan shavings. You can shave the cheese with a vegetable peeler. Sprinkle with the basil, and serve immediately.

INGREDIENTS

4 medium zucchini, cut into 1-inch slices

Juice of 1 lemon

2 tablespoons olive oil

Salt and freshly ground pepper

4-ounce piece of Parmesan cheese

2 tablespoons minced fresh basil

. . . .

SAUTÉED MUSHROOMS

Serves 4

INGREDIENTS

1½ pounds mixed
mushrooms (1 to 3
varieties)
2 tablespoons olive oil
Juice of ½ lemon
1 tablespoon unsalted
butter
Salt and freshly ground
pepper
2 tablespoons chopped
parsley
1 ounce grated Comté
cheese

1. Clean the mushrooms with paper towels (or clean pastry brush), and slice coarsely.

2. Heat the oil in a frying pan, add the lemon juice and mushrooms, and cook for a few minutes. Add the butter, and cook a few minutes more, until the liquid has evaporated. Season with salt and pepper to taste, and add the parsley.

3. Add the cheese, and cook a minute or so more, just until the cheese starts to melt. Mix gently, and serve immediately.

. . . .

SPINACH WITH RAISINS AND PINE NUTS

Serves 4

INGREDIENTS

2 pounds spinach
2 tablespoons olive oil

1. Wash the spinach and trim, if necessary.

2. Heat the oil in a large skillet. Sauté the raisins and pine nuts until golden, 1 to 2 minutes. Remove from the skillet, and set aside.

3. Add the spinach to the skillet. Season with salt and pepper to taste, cover, and cook over medium heat for 3 to 5 minutes or

until the spinach is wilted. Add the raisins and pine nuts, and toss constantly while cooking for 1 more minute. Serve immediately.

INGREDIENTS

2 tablespoons golden raisins

¼ cup pine nuts

Salt and freshly ground pepper

· ·

SPRING LAMB

In Europe, the Middle East, and North Africa, lambs have been sacrificed in connection with Christian, Jewish, and Muslim customs as long as those customs have existed (which suggests that people were offering up lambs in the cradle of civilization long before). I remember driving in Morocco—where lamb is the most commonly consumed red meat—during the feast commemorating the sacrifice of Isaac (known in Morocco as Eid el-Kebir) and seeing in village after village lambs hung by their feet with their necks sliced and blood dripping, in the ritually prescribed manner. In France, as elsewhere in Europe, spring lamb is associated with Easter, where it is a traditional dish, but it is now available year-round, not only because of demand-driven breeding but because of the contrariwise seasons of New Zealand and Australia, the world's largest exporters.

Since spring lambs are slaughtered at three to five months, they don't have the strong muttony flavor that sometimes puts off those unused to lamb. But the flavor, as well as the texture, can vary enormously. America produces lamb as good as can be found anywhere, though small local producers are the ones most likely to have taken the care to optimize the feed and hence the taste. Occasionally a fancy New York butcher has disappointed me, but the lamb man at the farmers' market can't afford to make mistakes.

CURRIED LAMB WITH EGGPLANT

Serves 4

INGREDIENTS

8 ounces yogurt

Juice of 2 lemons

2 tablespoons curry powder

1 pound lamb shoulder, deboned and cut in pieces

1 large eggplant, washed and diced

2 tablespoons olive oil

4 tablespoons minced shallots

1 cinnamon stick

1 star anise

2 tomatoes, diced

Salt and freshly ground pepper

4 tablespoons chopped fresh cilantro

1. With a fork, beat together 4 ounces of the yogurt, juice of 1 lemon, and 1 tablespoon curry. Pour over the lamb, and let marinate 2 to 3 hours in the refrigerator.

2. Steam the eggplant for 4 minutes, and set aside. Warm the oil over medium heat, and lightly brown the shallots. Add the cinnamon stick, star anise, and remaining curry, and cook for 1 minute. Stir in the eggplant and tomatoes. Season with salt and pepper to taste, and cook over low heat for 15 minutes.

3. Turn the broiler on, and cook the lamb with its marinade for 10 minutes, turning the meat a couple of times.

4. Combine the remaining yogurt and the juice of 1 lemon with the eggplant mixture, and cook for 5 minutes over medium-low heat. Add the cilantro. Serve the lamb (2 slices each) and eggplant.

RACK OF LAMB PERSILLADE

Serves 4 to 6

Easter Sunday was always my family's first taste of spring lamb (after we had the one made of angel food cake for breakfast), and Mamie *would always pick the simplest recipe (maybe that's why it was our favorite). Our third "lamb" of the day was actually a rereading of Saint-Exupéry's "lamb" chapter, in which the Little Prince asks,* "Dessine moi un mouton" *(draw me a sheep).*

1. Preheat the oven to 450 degrees.

2. Warm the oil in a skillet over medium-high heat. Add the garlic and shallots; stir for 10 seconds, add the bread crumbs and parsley, and stir for a minute more. Season with salt and pepper to taste, and set aside.

3. Season the lamb with salt and pepper, and arrange the racks in a baking pan. Pat the crumb mixture onto the meat sides and the fat of the lamb. Cook until a meat thermometer registers 130 degrees (for medium rare). Let the lamb stand for 5 minutes before carving. Cut the racks between bones into individual chops, 2 per person. Serve with peas.

INGREDIENTS

3 tablespoons olive oil

3 cloves garlic, peeled and minced

2 tablespoons minced shallots

¾ cup fresh bread crumbs

3 tablespoons minced parsley

Salt and freshly ground pepper

2 racks of lamb (4 ribs each)

Spring is full of harbingers, but none is more evocative of summer than the first great strawberries at market in late May or early June. As a child I liked to think that my father had planted the rows and rows of them in our garden with special affection, knowing them to be my favorite fruit. (I would have had him plant strawberry fields forever, if the song had then existed.) The ground around the plants was covered with straw so that each precious berry, after soaking up the vast amount of sunshine needed to ripen it, had its own cradle in which to fall, and therefore would need little or no washing. Papa grew two or three varieties with different ripening times to make the season last as long as possible. Those small- to medium-sized berries were moist and sweet and seductive. Alongside them, some of the big, red, photogenic California supermarket hybrids have as much claim to the name *strawberry* as today's steroid-enhanced athletes have to the mantle of Babe Ruth. Not surprisingly, ersatz strawberries have the same sort of nondescript taste and texture one finds in supermarket tomatoes: just enough to be discernible as the thing it's called, but ultimately only a taunt. They are overrefrigerated and served very cold—death for the flavor of most fruits.

Strawberries are versatile, so I try to observe the principle of *faire simple* (keep it simple), which should always be observed in preparing them. Shortcake can be delicious, but why overwhelm the taste of really good fruit? My favorite way to serve strawberries is sliced in a pretty dish with a tablespoon of mascarpone, crème fraîche, plain yogurt, fresh ricotta, whipped cream, or vanilla ice cream. A bit of freshly ground pepper can really pull the fruit and dairy flavors together, and today one can play with the huge variety of peppercorns.

For more elaborate desserts, I mostly avoid preparations like meringues that are heavy on sugar. As a rule, one should enjoy natural sweetness, and with good strawberries that's what you'll get. In Italy, great strawberries are served with just a squeeze of lemon, or sometimes a dash of fine aged balsamic vinegar. On the other hand, a nice *tarte sablée* covered with strawberries and a thin glaze of strawberry coulis is a platonically perfect confection—but I think of that more as a special treat than as the end of a meal. Desserts should be only as sweet as they need to be to cleanse the palate following the last savory course.

The sweetness of good strawberries can be channeled to help other fruits. I like to add a cup of strawberries a few minutes before I'm done making my rather acidic rhubarb compote. This I serve with yogurt or fresh ricotta, or with *fromage blanc,* a common marriage in French bistros during strawberry season.

For a further variation *aux fraises,* this on the sweeter side, try mixing a few fresh sliced strawberries with raspberries and serving them with a panna cotta or a custard: it's a nice contrast of textures, and though you're adding a bit of sweetness, you're still nowhere near the sugar surge of a strawberry shortcake.

RHUBARB-STRAWBERRY COMPOTE

Serves 4

Another simple, traditional recipe from childhood that has become the stuff of exquisite moments. The aroma of fresh fruit, so subtle and yet so intense, returns me to that bower where it seemed the strawberries would never end.

INGREDIENTS

⅓ cup sugar

¼ teaspoon cinnamon

1 tablespoon lemon juice

1 pound rhubarb, trimmed and cut into ½-inch pieces

½ cup strawberries, washed, drained, hulled, and sliced

1. Combine the sugar and cinnamon. Put the lemon juice into a saucepan with ¼ cup water and a third of the rhubarb, then sprinkle with the sugar-cinnamon mixture. Continue layering until all the rhubarb and sugar-cinnamon mixture is used up. Cover and cook gently over low heat until barely tender, 10 to 20 minutes.

2. Add the strawberries, and cook a few more minutes. Refrigerate until serving.

N.B. THE COMPOTE CAN ALSO BE EATEN AT ROOM TEMPERATURE AND IS A LOVELY ACCOMPANIMENT TO YOGURT (ABOUT 1 TABLESPOON PER 1/2 CUP OF YOGURT).

STRAWBERRY SOUP WITH MASCARPONE

Serves 4

1. Wash the strawberries. Gently pat dry, and hull all but 4 (reserve for decoration).

2. Mix the hulled strawberries, lemon juice, and sugar, and crush the strawberries slightly with a fork to release some juice.

3. In a separate bowl, beat the mascarpone with a whisk.

4. Pour the strawberry soup into martini glasses, and top with a dollop of mascarpone. Decorate each glass with a strawberry and a sprig of mint.

INGREDIENTS

1 pound strawberries

2 tablespoons lemon juice

2 tablespoons sugar

1 cup mascarpone

Fresh mint

. . . .

SPRINGING OUT OF THE CLOSET

Beyond cuisine, half the fun of the French woman's seasonal adjustment is the spring reorientation to life outdoors. And with that comes the seasonal adjustment of wardrobe, from heavy to light, from woolens to cottons, from darker to more vibrant colors. Some may take the view that color is "in" or it's "out" this year or that, but for me what nature is showing in a given season is far more influential than any designer's collection. With the freedom to unbundle oneself that warmer weather brings, spring is a great time to experiment as long as you *faîtes simple* with your look overall. I favor starting with clean lines and solid, often neutral separates—classic tees, polos, woven shirtings—of a quality that doesn't announce itself too loudly. A flattering, neat look can be had inexpensively by choosing clothes that fit, rather than constrain or billow. Trim, not tight, trousers, at a waist height dictated by your shape, not MTV.

Upon this neutral base I work the timeless custom of variation on a theme, namely, an arrangement of what have become my own signature accessories: necklace, sunglasses, and, above all, scarves. French women and scarves go together in people's minds. And French women generally effect their ever-changing self-styling with the cunning choice of accessories, most famously the scarf. Two of my most reliable ways to tie one in spring are the super simple classic kerchief and the more daring jacket scarf.

Classic Kerchief

This tie requires a square scarf and results in a V spread across your back with the knot hanging somewhere under your chin. A large scarf will flow over your shoulders; a small one creates the perfect spring look with a light, trimly cut crewneck sweater. You can also wear the scarf under the sweater for more of an ascot effect.

For a bit more glamour, in the evening, say, tie the scarf loosely and pull it down and around both shoulders to serve as a shawl. This is especially effective over low-cut dresses. Here's how:

1. Take the square scarf and fold it diagonally to form a triangle. Holding each end of the long length of the triangle, keep folding over the remaining point of the triangle until you have a band about two inches wide.

2. Still holding the long ends, drape the scarf around your neck and tie a square knot in front with a few inches of scarf flowering below the knot—that is, pull one of the long ends around the other, forming a loop through which to pass the first end. Tighten *comme tu veux*.

Mireille's Jacket Scarf

This requires a large, especially long rectangular scarf. I sometimes sew bands of silk onto the ends to add length and facilitate the knot.

1. Drape the scarf over your shoulders with one side hanging much longer than the other. For an average-sized woman that means one end should come just below your waist and the other just above your knees.
2. Crisscross the ends and wrap the longer end completely around your body until it meets the shorter end just above your hip. Tie with a simple knot.

The marvelous thing about this look is its versatility: it never comes out exactly the same twice. And depending on the scarf, it works as well for an outdoor café as for an outdoor cocktail with café society.

MUTABILITÉ

Ah, spring is here—but end it must, like all good things. I started this interlude with a bit of gushing about flowers as my dearest tokens of spring. Among those who don't suffer hay fever, I'm sure I would find not a few who feel likewise about nature's Technicolor cinema. Hardened indeed is the heart unmoved by the succession of crocuses, then daffodils, then tulips. The blooms on the almond trees of Provence in March. April's sacrament of the cherry blossoms in the American Northeast and Japan. And the dogwood in New York leading into May. What we sometimes forget to appreciate, on the other hand, is the satisfaction of their passing. If the cherry blossoms lasted for months, they would fast become a banality. Their mystery, their command of our attention, is exactly in proportion to their fleeting presence, what the Elizabethan poets obsessively referred to as *"mutabilitie,"* a Norman word (and still a French one). It was for this reason, I suppose, that van Gogh painted the irises in Provence rather than a still life of its more enduring lavender, however lovely that is.

A feature of our globalized marketplace is the constant availability of plant life out of its time; for a price, we can have the rarest orchids in our midst whenever. But this seems to me quite beside the point of flowers, if they may be said to have a point beyond their mere existence. What we appreciate, we appreciate in the fullness of time, though we can agreeably fool ourselves by protracting this a bit.

MENUS

"Le menu que je préfère (My favorite menu) / *c'est la chair de votre cou* (is the flesh of your neck)," sings Georges Brassens in *"J'ai rendez-vous avec vous"* ("I Have a Date with You"). Now that's a French menu. All about pleasure. Alas, the menus in this book, pure and simple, are not erotic. There's a place for that in healthy, balanced living, but I leave it to you to find it.

It goes without saying (or at least it should) that every day, every season, every menu for living should begin with the essence of life: a glass of water. If your tap water is unpalatable, as many are, find a bottled one you like and cultivate a taste that banishes those dubious drinks sweetened artificially or naturally. When starting her day, a French woman would no more neglect to have her glass of water than to dab a little perfume or eau de toilette on her neck.

Beyond water, bear in mind it is essential to have three meals. Your morning bread should be toasted (more digestible, and in France, yesterday's bread never goes to waste when there is always breakfast tomorrow). A sliver of butter is pure pleasure and much better for you than pseudo-fat substitutes like margarine, which should be tossed in the trash together with Crisco.

My three-meal-a-day menus provide a mix of proteins, carbohydrates, and fat, according to a rough ratio of 50–60/40–30/10 percent respectively. Remember you can be flexible—indulging a bit more here, paring back a bit there—but make sure that over the course of the week you find the balance. And enjoy! Eating is sensory, so eat with all five senses, and appreciate little experiences (of small portions and three bites) which produce through association and memory a gamut of emotions. Focus on the pleasurable ones and evade the destructive ones.

As they are subject to individual adjustments, my menu templates are equally suitable for maintaining a healthy weight and losing a few pounds following the principles of *French Women Don't Get Fat,* especially chapter 3 on short-term recasting. You'll need to tailor the menus somewhat to your own life.

The portions here are for little beings, like me, so if you are taller than average and proportionally heavier though not necessarily overweight, up your portions a bit. (Experiment with the 50 Percent Solution to see what satisfies you without causing weight gain.) And if that's not enough, incorporate a snack, yogurt being my first choice. (French women are the European champions, consuming on average 48.28 pounds of yogurt per year . . . on the way to not getting fat.)

As your sense of proportion evolves, feel free to make substitutions. I present a range of what I like, but you should suit yourself. If you prefer red wine with fish, go for it. If you don't like wine, you are missing one of the greatest foods on earth, but so be it. When I suggest noncaloric beverages I mean water or herbal tea (including green tea) or coffee. Try to limit other tea or coffee to no more than two servings a day, as the caffeine can make you hungry, especially on certain days of the month. It also dehydrates you, and the water in highly caffeinated beverages does *not* meet the requirement of drinking lots of plain water.

If you don't care for dried apricots have cranberries or whatever you like. Remember you can eat any good food in moderation . . . in three bites (so to speak). Small portions and variety are what matters. Learn to reduce at your pace by eating slowly and chewing well.

With soups especially, don't feel you have to follow the recipes to the letter. The same soup never tastes the same twice anyway. So don't panic if you are missing an ingredient: replace it with what you have on hand or prefer. (That goes for all dishes: you may, for instance, find that you prefer almonds over cashews with your spring asparagus. Nothing wrong with that.) I often throw in whatever I have in the fridge or find at the market. Be creative, bearing in mind the pleasures of mixing colors, though sometimes a delicious green soup needs no adornment.

For salads, I firmly believe the best dressing is a top-quality olive oil and vinegar (1 tablespoon vinegar for 3 tablespoons olive oil, an amount for 2 cups salad). If you need "spice" in your salad, add a bit of mustard to the dressing, and, of course, always plenty of fresh herbs. There is no such thing as a good bottled salad dressing.

Finally a few simple rules of thumb for easy portion approximation:

- For bread or chocolate, 1 ounce (that little scale is so useful).
- For cereal, ½ cup, ditto for milk. One cup if you've found your equilibrium.
- For rice, ⅓ cup cooked; potatoes, 3 ounces; pasta, ½ cup cooked (as a side dish; one cup as a main dish).
- For fruit, usually one piece or ½ cup is a portion. However, a whole banana, pear, grapefruit, or mango counts as two portions.

• A Week's Menu for Spring •

Breakfast

½ cup muesli
½ cup milk
½ cup strawberries
1 slice seven-grain bread,
    toasted and buttered
Coffee or tea

Lunch

2 cups spinach salad with
    mushrooms
Olive oil–vinegar dressing
2 ounces cheese of your
    choice
1 small roll
1 cup blueberries
Noncaloric beverage

Dinner

Calf's Liver with Greens
    (page 251)
½ cup sautéed potatoes
½ cup yogurt
2 clementines
1 glass red wine

Breakfast

2 prunes
½ cup yogurt with 1 table-
    spoon pecan granola and a
    drizzle of honey
1 tablespoon soy nuts
Coffee or tea

Lunch

Salade composée with hard-
    boiled egg, tuna, and
    haricots verts
Mustard-oil-vinegar dressing
1 slice whole wheat bread
1 pear
1 square chocolate
Noncaloric beverage

Dinner

Salmon with Sorrel
    (page 252)
½ cup Tagliatelle with
    Lemon (www.mireille
    guiliano.com)
2 slices baguette
Coffee *Petits Pots*
    (page 325)
1 glass red wine

• A Week's Menu for Spring •

Breakfast

½ cup bran flakes
½ cup milk
½ banana
1 slice rye bread, buttered
Coffee or tea

Lunch

Chicken breast with
   asparagus
½ cup yogurt
1 mango
Noncaloric beverage

Dinner

Roast Chicken with Endives
   (page 73)
Steamed Zucchini with Basil
   (page 77)
Strawberry Soup with
   Mascarpone (page 85)
1 glass white or red wine

Breakfast

½ cup freshly squeezed
   orange juice or 1 orange
1 soft-boiled egg
1 slice whole wheat bread,
   toasted and buttered
Coffee or tea

Lunch

Roast beef sandwich
Grated carrots with lemon-
   juice dressing
1 apple
Noncaloric beverage

Dinner

Spaghetti with Fiddlehead
   Ferns and Prosciutto
   (page 56–58)
Green salad
1 cup strawberries with a
   scoop of vanilla ice cream
1 glass red wine

• A Week's Menu for Spring •

Breakfast

1 slice boiled ham
½ cup yogurt
½ English muffin, toasted
   and buttered
1 kiwi
Coffee or tea

Lunch

Broccoli salad
Saumon à l'Unilatéral
   (www.mireilleguiliano
   .com)
Drizzle of olive oil on salmon
   and broccoli
1 slice bread
1 cup fruit salad
Noncaloric beverage

Dinner

Mackerel with Carrots and
   Leeks (page 71)
½ cup boiled potatoes
Fruit tart
1 glass red wine

Breakfast

2 ounces cheese
½ cup oatmeal with
   blueberries
⅓ cup milk
1 small brioche or slice of
   sourdough bread
Coffee or tea

Lunch

Leeks Mozzarella (page 68)
1 slice country bread
1 tangerine
Noncaloric beverage

Dinner

Steak
½ cup Mashed Potatoes
   (*Mamie's* Version) (page
   153)
Haricots Verts with
   Tomatoes (page 77)
Chocolate flan
1 glass red wine

• A Week's Menu for Spring •

Breakfast

½ cup fresh-squeezed orange
   juice or 1 orange
Asparagus and Cashew
   Omelet (page 50)
1 slice sourdough bread,
   toasted and buttered
Coffee or tea

Lunch

2 cups steamed vegetables
Olive oil–vinegar dressing
1 slice bread
½ cup yogurt
½ cup Rhubarb-Strawberry
   Compote (page 84)
Noncaloric beverage

Dinner

Curried Lamb with Eggplant
   (page 80)
½ cup pasta
Mixed green salad
1 cup strawberries with
   mascarpone
1 glass red wine

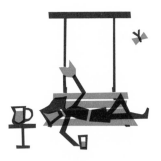

3

EN ÉTÉ: SUMMERTIME SMILES

And the livin' is easy. The French may have their much-ridiculed or envied six weeks of vacation—still but a fantasy for me, working in America, as for most of the world—but this is not to say that French women content themselves in summer with collapsing into a hammock and watching the cotton grow high. (Actually, we don't grow any.) In fact, most, myself included, seem to wake up a bit earlier and go to bed a bit later, taking full advantage of those precious few months of extra daylight. As long as I mind my equilibrium, I am full of energy, and it's never so easy to do as in summer.

Whether in New York, Paris, Provence, or elsewhere, the longest days are the most enlivening, the only limitation being heat, which can become oppressive—even in Provence. There are places where the broiling, humid outdoors of summer is simply unbearable; in such places, summer can seem a kind of winter, an interval of harshness from which to take refuge. (It's no coincidence that summer and winter are the seasons that are also verbs. No one goes somewhere else "to autumn.") I do not dispute the discomfort of people in these places, but to some degree, it is another way we have become victims of modern conveniences and modern expectations. Even in places where summer seems quite pleasant, people spend too much of it in an air-conditioned bubble as the standard for comfort has changed. As for those places that verge on the tropical in summer, there is no debating the matter. In Houston, for instance, a fascinating and vibrant town despite having won in 2005 the dubious distinction of the fattest city in America (supplanted in 2006 by Chicago—likewise a place of sometimes unbearable extremes of temperature), winter is mild while summer is harsh, with people scurrying from car to mall to car to house, if not fleeing to Colorado. (Some of the most elaborate "swankiendas" even have air-conditioned backyards.)

It's sad to imagine summer as an event to be escaped, but in more and more places it has become that. It occurs to me that we used to make less evasive accommodations to nature, such as screened-in verandas, fans, and plenty of lemonade; in the course of an agreeably slower but still active way of life, we would tolerate a bit of sweat (not the social abomination Madison Avenue makes it seem). I don't think it's coincidence that the fattening of America has tracked with the spread of climate control and television. We cannot go back to the way things were, but the goal should still be to seek out the season as one can, and not only during vacations. Summer is the interval of peak experience, a state of being and a state of mind, and properly speaking, not a time we should be getting fat.

For me summer registers with evenings and weekends spent outdoors whenever conditions permit. Outdoor food markets crop up in summer like mushrooms after a storm. The variety of seasonal produce—fresh berries, vegetables whose brilliant color announces the nutrients packed within (nature's food labeling), fresh and fragrant herbs, and gorgeous flowers—is truly an embarrassment of riches. I find walking among the market stalls a superb way to relax, a fine occasion to see or meet friends, talk to farmers, and drink in the blue sky and the sun—protected, of course, with SPF 15, sunglasses, and a hat. French women are very careful about the sun, especially where their faces are concerned, for nothing adds years to the face or hands like too many youthful days spent unprotected in solar radiance. Saying this, I must note that enjoyment of the sun brings out the American tendency toward unhealthy extremism, and not only in Americans. Devoted readers of health and beauty magazines, ever on the lookout for new products with astronomical SPFs, seem obsessed with going anywhere *but* toward the light. Others take the arrival of summer sun as the occasion to roast like *poulets* on a spit, heedless of common sense, let alone medical fact. Raising the bar for what constitutes a healthy glow, they compel their more vampirish sisters to slather on the tanner-in-a-tube, which leaves virtually all complexions some shade of cantaloupe. We need a little *bon sens* here: The sun is essential for our synthesis of vitamin D, without which our bones would turn to coral. So you should make sure to get some, but limit your exposure (a burn can occur in ten minutes without protection), take extra pains to protect your face and hands, and neither a sun worshipper nor a vampire be.

Summer dress is light dress, often white and light colors, mostly cotton. But don't forget that on the hottest days in hotter climes more cover can keep you cooler than less, to say nothing of protecting unnoticed body parts from sun damage and far worse. In a French city you'll see few locals over the age of twelve wearing shorts, and decent "cover" is the norm (except perhaps in Saint-Tropez). I lose the heels in favor of lower sandals or espadrilles—a classic style that never disappears from the maritime regions of France and all along the Mediterranean. With regular cycling and swimming, two of my favorite activities, I wind up washing my hair too often for a cut that requires a lot of styling. Summer is a good time to *faire simple* with your hair, although you shouldn't ignore the necessity of special care. Hot climates, whether dry or humid, do wreak havoc on both hair and skin. As in winter, the need to moisturize is great. For the hair a thick shea butter conditioner is advisable several times a week, depending on how naturally dry your hair might be. Frizz is proportional to dryness: need I say more? Before moisturizing, I rinse my hair with cold water to which I've added a teaspoon of vinegar or the juice of a lemon, as my mother taught me to do: this will make it shinier than expensive products will. I also like to rinse my body in the shower with cold water; it's good for the circulation. These are cold-water beauty routines that are actually a good year-round habit, but if you didn't grow up in northern France, you might find it easier to start them in summer. The same might be said for my morning ritual of putting an ice cube or two in a facecloth (to avoid breaking capillaries) and gently stroking my face, especially around the eyes. I do this right after I've had my day's first glass of water; the day's first one is vital, also regardless of season.

So, creams, sun protection, and moisturizers for hair and body are part of the seasonal toolbox. But in summer, makeup too takes a holiday. Go light, without foundation for the chic, un-made-up look of Parisians. Put on some sunscreen, and let your skin breathe. A mask is a good idea. My mother had two wonderful ones for summer: strawberry (mash a few strawberries and mix together with ½ teaspoon of honey and ½ teaspoon of Vaseline moisturizer. Apply to your whole face; after fifteen minutes, rinse off) and cucumber (mix a few cucumber slices with 2 tablespoons of yogurt and apply to your face and eyes. Cover with a wet cloth; after fifteen minutes, rinse off). As for fragrances, I vary them by season, too, in spring and summer preferring eau de toilette to perfume, light florals and refreshing citrusy scents, nothing too complex or heady.

High-maintenance looks take time away from what ought to be the most routinely active season of the year, when the urge to be outside keeps us on the go and even in America work does slow down a bit. If you do not seize the day, if you become a summer hibernator, you will be working against the season's natural mechanism for preserving your weight equilibrium. Here it is *en bref:* Summer gives us a bounty of super-satisfying flavors, which, if consciously savored, steer us clear of offenders. The heat of summer is not conducive to overeating, as the body craves food rich in readily digestible energy and much-needed water and electrolytes. It feels great to be out and about, so routine exertion is easy, especially if we make a point of doing our walking early in the morning and evening. The urge to participate in summer fun also creates occasions for sports, however undignified: many who would never claim any prowess at softball can be dragged onto the field in the spirit of summer. Don't be proud—go with it. I'm hardly a great swimmer, but whenever possible, I avail myself of one of the most joint-friendly and meditative of all activities. There is much to do because it's fun. Thus not getting fat becomes a fringe benefit rather than the end in itself.

On Saturdays in summer when I was child, my mother would serve us a cold lunch on the shaded terrace overlooking the garden. The day would have started and ended, as it still does, with a tall glass of water. She took pains to be sure that we were never dehydrated; there would be a full pitcher, frequently refilled, all day long. Mother would bring a baguette, a couple of cheeses, some salami or ham, while I, with a visiting friend or two, would go to the garden to pluck a few tomatoes, some radishes, and some fresh lettuce (we would rinse our pickings at the garden tap, never stepping foot in the house). That labor was rewarded later with free, exclusive access to the berry bushes; after eating our sandwiches, slowly of course, there was a digestive pause, and then we were each handed a little bowl with which to forage. It's as if my mother knew we would otherwise just crouch there putting berries into our mouths without a thought for the others waiting at the table. We did, however, manage to make it back with bowlfuls for them, too. Afterward, we'd just sit and talk lazily till midafternoon. Even with the doors and windows arranged for a cross breeze, it was simply too hot at midday to sit indoors, much less to exert oneself outside. Evenings were when we played, and on the longest days it would be light out until ten.

We were left to our own devices in the big garden. Mid-afternoon, one of our neighbors, Madame Regnaud, would often come with a new children's book she was reading to her grandchildren, and she would read us a story or two in the shade of the terrace; with our eyes shut, we could hear nothing but her voice over the happy chatter of the birds. *Mamie* would reappear around *le 4 heures* for the afternoon refreshment, not a *goûter* (snack) but glasses of lemonade she had made fresh, mindful of our need for water, especially in summer. It was neither tart nor especially sweet. Looking back, what strikes me most is not how much this scene resembles one from the nineteenth century but how remote it seems from the twenty-first. In fact, the pace of lifestyle change has picked up dramatically within only the past few decades. Unfortunately, we seem to have taken little care to compensate for the things subtracted. Most children today would choose the air-conditioned family room, with the latest version of PlayStation by the light of the plasma, over sitting around outside in summer's heat. Needless to say, it's a different sort of conditioning in terms of comfort and pleasure. As for me, I'm quite grateful that to this day, given my druthers, on a Saturday afternoon in summer I can be found outside in a shady refuge amid flowers, a book in hand, a glass of lemony water or cooled herbal tea of mint or basil nearby.

Of course, we're not kids anymore and can't all spend the whole summer as we might like. Nearly all of us with jobs indoors must spend most of the day in the air-conditioned bubble I mentioned. On workdays, the heat seems particularly uncomfortable because it can defeat our efforts at neat professional presentation. And we must devise accommodations for passing from the sultry street into the meat locker that most offices and shops and restaurants—all public places, really—become in summer. And this is the case now even in some parts of Europe, which was slower to accept air-conditioned living. The simplicity of French women's self-styling is never handier than in summer. I often recommend starting the season with a uniform in mind. A few pairs of flattering trousers, a skirt, and fine cotton T-shirts. Buy the nicest you can. It's better to have a few good pieces than two weeks' worth of shoddy clothes. The shirts—mercerized or knitted cotton of good quality gives you a base of simplicity without looking slovenly—should be easily washed and ironed. Simple is best, though a few buttons, a ribbed weave, or subtle piping announces that you are not sporting Fruit of the Loom. J. Crew and Banana Republic are just two of the retailers offering such basics online at a good price. The trousers, if of a light tropical wool, can be hung in a steamy bathroom or pressed with a not-too-hot iron several times before you need to take them to the dry cleaner (dry cleaning wears out fibers and makes new clothes look worn, so do it sparingly). If the trousers are linen, their wrinkling is perfectly stylish. With their nice tees and trousers or simple sheath dresses, French women, as I shared, create their different looks with accessories.

The jewelry does not require a trip to Cartier. I have a string of chunky wooden beads I bought in the souk in Marrakesh, and they lend a very sophisticated touch to a tee and trousers. This year white beads were all the rage and didn't need to be made of ivory to look elegant. (Who would be so cruel to Babar, anyway?) You could buy a modish ornament at a fancy boutique, but often a look-alike piece from some other emporium—or even a street vendor—will create the same effect for a lot less money. (Makes sense, since the more determinedly fashionable the look, the less likely you'll want to embrace it next season.) With jewelry, less is most definitely more. If you have a choker making a strong statement, you don't need elaborate earrings—de trop. To be in fashion as well as stylish (the latter being a more evolved and personal state of being, a mind-set as much as a look), limit yourself to an element or two—a color, a shape of handbag—that signals you are not totally oblivious to the pages of *Vogue* and *Elle*. Remember: French women do not "buy the mannequin." Nor do they adhere militantly to the haute bourgeois ideal of always looking totally "done." They do one part uniform, one part fashion statement, and one part strictly idiosyncratic and personal. The specific choices are yours.

This way, you should navigate the street chicly in summer. But what of the air-conditioned bubble? Don't blow money on trendy glad rags if you haven't invested in a classic crewneck cardigan in light cashmere, if you can afford it. It is always elegant, can be draped over the shoulders or folded into a tote, and may save you from hypothermia at your desk. A good cashmere cardigan, occasionally hand washed and combed for pilling, can last for years. Next summer you can start building your collection, adding a new sweater each year. (A little quality goes a long way—you needn't bankrupt yourself buying en masse.) Start with a neutral color you can wear all the time.

Another means of deliverance from the artificial Arctic is the scarf, which perhaps sounds like the last thing one would need in summer. In fact, like a cunning string of beads, a neckerchief can dress up and lend individuality to a simple tee-and-skirt ensemble while taking the chill off, too. When not wrapped in one, French women keep the scarf handily tied to the handles of their handbags. This is part of the effortless look commonly called BCBG (*bon chic, bon genre*)—half style, half attitude, meant to channel the *bien dans sa peau* spirit if not taken to fussy extremes. I tend to wear cotton, muslin, or chiffon scarves in summer, and I tend to wear them differently than in other seasons.

Belt Scarf

One of the easiest ways to bring a scarf along to lunch or a shopping excursion is to wear it as a belt, unfurling it across your shoulders if you feel cold. For this you will need an oblong scarf.

1. Fold and refold lengthwise until you have created a band about five inches wide.
2. Wrap the scarf about your hips and tie with a square knot or bow. The bow side of the belt will be crimped to about three inches wide.
3. Slide the bow to one hip, and spread the band downward on the opposite hip to create an isosceles triangle with its point at the bow.

Hip Wrap

A chic way to carry a large, square scarf.

1. Fold it diagonally in half. Wrap it around your waist with the triangle pointing downward behind you.

2. Tie the two ends in the front with a square knot. Tug the two sides down over your hips.

Stole

The simplest way—and a very common one—to wear a scarf is to transform your belt scarf or hip wrap into a stole.

1. Take the unfolded scarf and simply drape it evenly over your shoulders. The ends should fall into the crooks of your elbows.
2. Still cold? Pull one end to lengthen it and toss the longer side over the opposite shoulder for a double layer of fabric.

Pool or Beach Scarf Skirt or Dress

Long gone are the days of bronzing myself on the Riviera with teenage abandon (back when we still believed the sun could do us nothing but good). Today, I wrap myself a bit when wearing a bathing suit in the company of strangers—except in the water, of course. And while a whole retail sector has sprung up to furnish "cruisewear," I find a lightweight scarf can cover it, and me. I wear it as a skirt with a one-piece, as a dress with a two-piece. You'll need a large, square scarf for a skirt and an even larger one, square or rectangular, for a dress. With a scarf wrap you can always make a quick exit from the beach to lunch without going indoors to change.

For the skirt:
1. Fold the square in half diagonally.
2. Flip or fold the long length into a little belt or band, wrap around your waist, and tie over your hips or behind your back. Adjust for length. *Et voilà.*

For the dress:

1. Drape the open scarf across your back; pass an end under each arm, and tie a tight knot in front.
2. Fold the upper edge of the scarf inward to conceal the knot. Pull down on that part to give the neckline a slight V for an illusion of constructedness.

Summer being the traditional time for *les vacances* when I was younger, it also meant going away somewhere, whether for a few weeks to my grandmother's house in rural Alsace, a summer job in Austria, or relief work in Yugoslavia. Whatever the itinerary, the point was to be closer to the season, not to escape it. I came to the custom of a beach holiday fairly late, first on the Riviera (not as glamorous for French people as it sounds to Americans), then as an exchange student on Nantucket with my adoptive American family. The latter was a much more exotic experience, in terms of both landscape (*sandy* beaches, not the norm in France) and social anthropology. There is a point to travel that is very much like the point of seasonality: it helps our mental organization of time, breaking it up, and makes our overall experience seem fuller. As nature designed us, our senses perk up in any unfamiliar setting, trying to take everything in, feeding information directly to our so-called reptilian cortex, a vestige of a time before we had mastered our surroundings and needed to be watchful for dangers and potential meals. For this reason, Chianti at home doesn't taste the way it tastes in Tuscany. Lavender bundles even at the Paris markets don't smell like the air in Provence. The play of the light in Miami is one glory, the play of the light in the Alps another. A change of scene is good for us because it gives all our senses a new world of stimuli to react to.

But not everyone seems as clued in to the importance of this phenomenon to overall health. While the serenity of the beach makes it a vacation destination I love—nothing is more meditative than the sea, and a walk along the edge of the surf is the most pleasant of exertions—I have met many women of all ages who think of it as an occasion to lose consciousness. "I just want to veg" is an expression I've heard countless times from hardworking people explaining their beach holidays from mindfulness. True, modern living gives us too much to think about, and the world is changing faster than we can make sense of it. The antidote, however, may not be to stop thinking but to think of something else. Being lulled into oblivion by tropical drinks and drowsy heat may not furnish nearly as much rest or renewal as we can be tempted to imagine. It's just a respite. Occasionally, *ça suffit* (it's enough). In general, though, time away is better spent immersing oneself in something different—a landscape, a culture, even a different language, and *bien sûr* a different cuisine. You don't need to trek through the Atlas Mountains or bobsled to the Arctic. But a sense of place and time—of journey—is vital for me. My years feel fuller for having been marked by incredible moments in unimposing places: an out-of-the way little restaurant in southern Sicily, a small temple near Kyoto, an inn with an aspiring chef in the Massif Central. In such circumstances, gluttony never occurs to you. There you simply feel free.

As I say, it doesn't have to be exotic, just consistently stimulating. For the past fifteen years, since we first started to rent a house in Provence and especially now that we own one, summer has increasingly been centered on one place. But it's a place of such intensities that for us it remains an undiscovered country: the heat, the crickets, the lavender, the most bountiful markets, the most mesmeric sunsets—truly a world full of inspiration. Provence is, in a way, my summer state of mind, the dream of perfect abundance and peace that abides with me year-round. It's not hard getting friends to visit us, although some wonder why I do it so regularly, since taking good care of people can be hard work. Actually, I find it stimulating to help other people relax. My only demand is that they surrender all handheld devices—at least telephonic ones—when they cross our threshold. Some city friends really have a hard time and truly don't know how to relax. But once the mind is engaged, once we call their attention to this little wonder and that small miracle, the spirit follows.

Summer weekend meals at home, whether in town or country, whether à deux or with friends, are as simple as it gets with us. The fresher the produce, the less you need to do to it. So much of cooking was invented to make something edible out of something unpalatable as found in nature, especially at those times of year when nature offers the least. This necessity has no bearing in summer, when there is plenty to eat raw, and even more that requires only the lightest culinary touch. Besides, who wants to fuss in the heat?

Very little is gastronomically out of bounds, especially if it can go on the grill. The scope of grillable food has been deliciously expanded by inventive chefs in recent years. We love grilled vegetables as appetizers; fish, meat, and chicken are a dream; and grilled peaches for dessert are simply heaven. (We haven't yet devised a barbecue version of baked Alaska, but

Edward is working on it.) Picnics are another great way to *faire simple:* some cheese and a *saucisson* plus some wine and bread can seem a feast in a field or under a tree, especially after you've walked around and let the surroundings do a number on your senses. At last, though they come first for French women, soups—the indispensable staple for all seasons—have a special part to play in summer. They're the easiest way to release the fleeting intensities of seasonal produce, a light and digestible but extremely satisfying and versatile meal. (If you work at it, you can almost manage never to make the same soup twice.) Most important, they help keep us hydrated in the months when we quite naturally sweat. A hot soup, like hot tea, can cool you off, but a cold soup sometimes seems more palatable; though the range of possibilities may be smaller, when a cold soup is good, it's great.

Many people are surprised by how easily soup can be made, without the bother of an endlessly simmering pot, provided that you have set aside half a day during those long winter months to make some fresh stock, which can be frozen, then thawed as needed. After serving chicken to guests, I often throw the carcass into a stockpot with mirepoix (diced root vegetables and bacon) while Edward serves the dessert; they're finishing one meal, I'm starting the next. (If that soothing activity is too much for you, take heart: simple and delicious soup can be made using water, with no stock at all or, with a little effort, you can find good-quality store-bought stock.) Many vegetables you regularly cook—roasting, grilling, boiling them, whatever suits the particular type—can then be puréed in a mill with a bit of stock or water. This mixture is an excellent base upon which to start inventing with your favorite spices and herbs, perhaps finishing with a dollop of yogurt, a piece of soft cheese, or a powdering of the grated hard stuff. The starch in the puréed vegetables gives the soup body, making unnecessary the cream or eggs of a bisque or a velouté, as well as the attendant fuss.

SOUPS

COLD CUCUMBER SOUP

Serves 4

My Provençal friends call this soup Gazpacho à la Mireille, although it lacks the acidity of its Spanish namesake—something of an acquired taste (as we both are). I love to serve it for lunch on hot, dry summer days. Sometimes I purée it before chilling. The cucumber is, like the leek, a mild diuretic, rich in potassium and low in sodium; both help flush out the toxins. The shrimp provides protein; with a slice of baguette or brown bread and some fresh fruit for dessert, the dish makes for a deliciously well-rounded summer lunch in the shade, listening to the cigales *(crickets), or your children chatter.*

1. Cut the cucumbers in half lengthwise, scoop out the seeds with a teaspoon, and cut into 1-inch pieces. Sprinkle with salt, and let stand 10 minutes. Drain and pat dry.

INGREDIENTS

2 8-inch cucumbers (about 1 pound), peeled

Salt and freshly ground pepper

INGREDIENTS

1 cup cold milk (regular or
2 percent)

1 cup yogurt

Juice of 1 lemon

4 tablespoons minced mint
leaves

½ cup shrimp, peeled,
deveined, and cooked

⅓ cup mint leaves for
garnish

2. Mix the cucumber with the milk. Add the yogurt, lemon juice, and minced mint, and season with salt and pepper to taste. Serve sprinkled with the shrimp and decorated with mint leaves.

· ·

GREEN SOUP

Serves 4

My friend Jacqueline is nuts about greens and is always coming up with new recipes. Here's her latest, which I love.

INGREDIENTS

2 tablespoons olive oil

2 leeks, white parts only,
thinly sliced

2½ cups green beans cut
into 2-inch pieces

2½ cups small broccoli
florets

2 medium zucchini, sliced

5 cups vegetable stock
(or water)

1. Warm the oil in a pot over medium heat, and cook the leeks for a few minutes. Add the green beans and cook for 5 minutes, stirring occasionally. Add the broccoli, zucchini, and vegetable stock. Bring to a boil, then reduce the heat and simmer for 20 to 25 minutes. When the vegetables are tender, put through a vegetable mill.

2. Return the milled vegetables to the pot. Season with salt and pepper to taste, add the milk, and cook, stirring, over medium heat for 10 minutes more. Sprinkle with parsley, and serve.

INGREDIENTS

Salt and freshly ground pepper

2½ cups milk (regular or 2 percent)

4 tablespoons minced parsley

. . . .

BEET SOUP

Serves 4

For taste and texture, nothing beats beets in a salad or soup. I make this soup in advance and serve it right out of the refrigerator. I ask my guests if they want theirs à la vieille Russie (traditionally served hot with a swirl of sour cream) or the French way.

1. Combine the beets and yogurt, and stir well. Add the shallots, garlic, and cumin. Season with salt and pepper to taste, and mix well. Refrigerate for at least 2 hours.

2. Serve in chilled soup bowls after correcting seasoning and sprinkling with the dill.

INGREDIENTS

1 pound red beets, cooked and cubed

1 cup yogurt

2 tablespoons minced shallots

1 teaspoon minced garlic

Pinch of cumin

Salt and freshly ground pepper

2 tablespoons dill

. . . .

COLD FENNEL SOUP

Serves 4

My friend Christine is a fennel freak (not to be confused with fenugreek), and I daresay I am too. All summer long, I eat it raw or cooked, by itself or in combination, as in this soup. In Indian restaurants, you'll often find the seeds in a little bowl as you are leaving—like parsley, they are nature's great breath freshener. Christine makes the soup using small, young, tender fennel bulbs. Being in Provence, she adds the local brousse cheese, *but I have made it in New York using fresh ricotta with comparable results.*

INGREDIENTS

5 cups vegetable stock (or water)

1 pound fennel bulbs, cleaned and chopped

4 ounces ricotta

1 tablespoon olive oil

2 tablespoons lemon juice

Salt and freshly ground pepper

4 tablespoons minced parsley

Pinch of paprika

1. Bring the stock to a boil. Add the fennel pieces, and simmer for 20 minutes. Put the fennel and stock through a blender or vegetable mill using a blade with smaller holes. Let cool, and refrigerate for 2 hours.

2. Add the ricotta, oil, and lemon juice to the chilled soup. Mix well, and season with salt and pepper to taste. Serve in soup dishes, garnishing with the parsley and paprika.

SUMMER-VEGETABLE SOUP WITH CHEESE

Serves 4

Those females in my family, with their tireless imaginations, would find no end of ways to slip in an extra food group, turning a soup into a more nutritionally balanced meal. Why make a béchamel when protein is so easy to add in the form of a little cheese? With good bread and some fruit, how could you want more?

1. Warm the oil in a large pot over medium heat, and sauté the onion and shallots until translucent. Add the potatoes, carrots, sweet pepper, and water. Bring to a boil, then lower the heat and simmer for 15 to 20 minutes.

2. Sprinkle with the feta, and add the lemon juice. Season with salt and pepper to taste, and serve.

INGREDIENTS

2 tablespoons olive oil

1 onion, minced

2 shallots, minced

1 pound potatoes, peeled and cubed

1 pound carrots, peeled and sliced

1 sweet pepper (green, yellow, or red), seeds removed, sliced into 2-inch strips

6 cups water

6 ounces feta cheese

1 tablespoon lemon juice

Salt and freshly ground pepper

COLD CARROT SOUP

Serves 4

INGREDIENTS

3 cups water

1½ pounds carrots, peeled

½ cup Idaho potatoes, peeled

1⅓ cups cold milk (regular or 2 percent)

3 tablespoons minced basil

Salt and freshly ground pepper

1. In a large pot, bring the salted water to a simmer, and cook the carrots and potatoes until tender, about 20 minutes. Cool, and put through a vegetable mill. Refrigerate for at least 2 hours.

2. Add the milk and basil, and mix well. Season with salt and pepper to taste, and serve very cold.

· ·

MELON SOUP

Serves 4

As refreshing as it gets, and a delicious tease for those with a sweet tooth.

INGREDIENTS

1 quart water

3 ounces raw almonds, finely ground

2 egg yolks

2 tablespoons sour cream

Salt and freshly ground pepper

1 melon

1. In a large pot, bring the water to a boil, then add the ground almonds. Bring back to a boil over low heat, then turn off the heat, cover, and leave 15 minutes to infuse. Filter through a fine sieve.

2. In a large bowl, beat the egg yolks with the sour cream. Add the warm infusion a little at a time, stirring all the while. Allow the mixture to cool. Season with salt and pepper to taste.

3. Cut the melon in half and remove the seeds. Cut the flesh into small dice, and add to the soup. Serve with a garnish of dill and almond slivers.

INGREDIENTS

2 tablespoons chopped dill

1 ounce almond slivers, toasted

. . . .

VICHYSSOISE
(COLD LEEK AND POTATO SOUP)
Serves 4

1. Melt the butter in a large pot over medium heat. Add the leeks and onion, and cook for 10 minutes over medium-low heat. Add the potatoes, then the stock, and bring to a boil. Lower the heat, and simmer for 35 minutes, partly covered.

2. Put through a vegetable mill (and then, if you want a very thin soup, through a chinois). Return the liquid to the pot, and season with salt and pepper to taste. Bring back to a boil, and whisk in the sour cream.

3. When the soup has cooled, refrigerate for at least 6 hours. Serve cold, preferably in coffee cups, and sprinkled with dill.

INGREDIENTS

2 tablespoons unsalted butter

4 leeks, white parts only, minced

1 onion, peeled and minced

½ pound potatoes, peeled and diced

1 quart chicken stock

Salt and freshly ground pepper

2 ounces (¼ cup) sour cream

Dill for garnish

N.B. A VERSION MADE BY AN ITALIAN FRIEND IN PROVENCE REPLACES LEEKS WITH ZUCCHINI (REDUCE COOKING TIME BY 10 MINUTES) AND USES MASCARPONE INSTEAD OF SOUR CREAM AND BASIL INSTEAD OF DILL. *ASSOLUTAMENTE DELICIOSA.*

French women and virtually all foodies rave about tomatoes in season. If you've heard nothing else about the magic of seasonality, you have almost surely heard (dozens of times) that the difference between a fresh tomato in season and a supermarket tomato in December (or July, for that matter) is night and day. A specimen of the real thing can seem like a meal; the common counterfeit defames even a BLT.

If daffodils and strawberries tell me it's spring, nothing says summer like a sunflower and the red of a perfectly ripe tomato. Why do we wax rhapsodic over this most common vegetable, which everyone learns and then forgets is a fruit? (Important distinction, since you might *par hasard* put one in the refrigerator, and nobody would do that with a ripe fruit, would they? Of course not.) The thing about the tomato, my favorite fruit that isn't a strawberry, is that it actually *is* rather like a strawberry: of all fruits, these two have been optimally designed to capture the energy of the sun and turn it into some of the best eats on earth.

Now, do a tomato wrong—pick it unripe, ship it north, set it to brood on a supermarket shelf—and you'll get exactly what you deserve: a potato with a little extra lycopene. Actually, I'm being grossly unfair to the potato, but tubers will have their moment in winter. For now, however, it's summer, and in summer you should permit tomatoes to do their thing: let the sunshine in. The best tomatoes (and basil, for that matter) I ever tasted were in Puglia, Italy. French women brook no chauvinism where produce is concerned: best is best. Maybe it was the local combination of heat and dryness, but the intensity of the flavors was unequaled, and the Italians know a good thing when they taste it; on the autostrada near the tomato canning plant in Avellino I've seen caravans of trucks in summer laden with tomatoes on their way to becoming sauce. (By the way, a good tomato sauce in can or jar is worth ten rotten tomatoes on the shelf: come winter, it's the best way to keep this sacrament of summer in your life and profit from its matchless concentration of nutrients. And, oh, the taste!)

An old friend of mine has tomatoes every day for breakfast during the season, which is basically the summer months, wherever he is. I suspect that, being an older gent, he's not only hooked on the taste but wants the lycopene, a known prostate-cancer inhibitor. A cousin who's never had a prostate, however, also likes tomatoes for her breakfast. She used to make her own *confiture de tomates,* a jam of seedless tomatoes (though she would keep the skin), puréeing them with a pinch of sugar and adding a vanilla bean before transferring it to a sterile jar. At breakfast, she has her slice of bread with the confit smeared on it, hold the butter. Tell me it's not a fruit!

In New York, I could not survive summer without New Jersey beefsteak tomatoes, a large variety with a distinctive flavor. Brought to market fresh from the farm, they are delicious sliced and served with slivers of mozzarella, a light dressing, and fresh basil—what the Italians call an *insalata Caprese,* though it's enjoyed many places far from Capri. I apply the same recipe in Provence, where the day's main meal is lunch (as often as not followed by an afternoon dodge-the-heat siesta, then, toward sunset, an outing for some illicit raspberry picking from the communal bushes along the road). Late dinner, served outdoors, often consists of no more than a tomato salad with some nice country bread to mop up the juice and dressing, fresh goat cheese, and various fresh fruits for dessert. Sounds like not much? Trust me, no one leaves the table unsatisfied.

A real treat for us tomato heads is an entire meal based on them. To this day the only chef I have found who can truly pull it off is Christian Étienne in Avignon. I have sent friends to him who liked it so much, they had to go back the same week. The versatility of tomatoes is such that you can contemplate even a multicourse meal centered on them without a chance of boredom. And no American ever sees a tomato dessert coming!

MIREILLE'S SIMPLE TOMATO SALAD
Serves 4

INGREDIENTS

6 tomatoes
1½ teaspoons coarse salt
4 tablespoons olive oil
Freshly ground pepper
4 tablespoons basil cut into chiffonade

1. Slice the tomatoes ¼ inch thick, and spread equally over 4 flat dishes. Sprinkle with the salt, and let stand for 20 minutes. (This is the trick that extracts flavor.) Then remove excess water with paper towels.

2. Drizzle each dish of tomatoes with 1 tablespoon of the oil, and season with pepper to taste. Sprinkle with the basil, and serve with country bread to dunk into that delicious juice and clean the plate.

OPTIONAL: SOME PEOPLE LIKE TO ADD A DROP OR TWO OF VINEGAR OR SOME FINELY SLICED ONIONS.

· ·

SWEET-AND-SOUR FRUIT-AND-VEGETABLE SALAD

Serves 4

1. Steam the haricots verts for 8 minutes, and set aside.

2. Steam the corn for 3 minutes; cool, then slice the kernels off the cob with a sharp knife.

3. Sprinkle the avocado slices with the lemon juice.

4. For the dressing, put the mustard, salt and pepper to taste, and vinegar in a bowl, and stir well. Add both oils, and whisk well.

5. Put all the fruits and vegetables in a serving bowl, pour the dressing over, and toss gently.

INGREDIENTS

½ pound fresh haricots verts

2 ears of corn

1 avocado, cut into thin slices

Juice of 1 lemon

1 teaspoon Meaux mustard

Salt and freshly ground pepper

2 tablespoons red wine vinegar

3 tablespoons olive oil

3 tablespoons sunflower oil

1 head lettuce, torn into leaves, rinsed, and dried

1 grapefruit, peeled, sliced, and pith removed

10 ounces fresh pineapple, cubed

ORECCHIETTE WITH TUNA AND ZUCCHINI

Serves 4

INGREDIENTS

12 ounces (about 4 cups) orecchiette

2 medium zucchini, thinly sliced

1 tablespoon unsalted butter or olive oil

2 cloves garlic, peeled and minced

1 pound cherry tomatoes, halved

1 6-ounce can tuna in olive oil

4 tablespoons olive oil

Salt and freshly ground pepper

2 tablespoons chopped fresh basil

1. Bring 8 cups of salted water to a rolling boil in a large pot. Cook the orecchiette according to package directions.

2. Place the zucchini in a large serving bowl. Drain the pasta over the bowl, and let the zucchini stand in hot cooking water 2 minutes to soften. Drain, and return zucchini to bowl.

3. Melt the butter (or heat the 1 tablespoon oil) in a large skillet. Sauté the garlic and tomatoes over medium heat until softened. Remove from heat. Add the tuna. Toss with the pasta, zucchini, and drizzle the oil over all. Season with salt and pepper to taste, and sprinkle with the basil. Serve immediately.

· ·

RED MULLET WITH SPINACH EN PAPILLOTE

Serves 4

INGREDIENTS

2 teaspoons olive oil

1 pound spinach, washed and dried

1. Preheat the oven to 300 degrees.

2. Cut 8 pieces of parchment paper (or aluminum foil) into squares large enough to cover each fish fillet and leave a 2-inch

border all around. Lightly brush 4 squares of the paper with oil.

3. In the center of an oiled square, layer a quarter of the spinach, 1 tablespoon of the crème fraîche, 2 fillets, 1 teaspoon of the shallots, and 2 slices of lime. Season with salt and pepper to taste.

4. Place the remaining parchment squares on top of the fillets and fold up the edges to form packets. Simply double folding each of the four sides is enough to seal each packet. Put the *papillotes* on a baking sheet, and bake in the preheated oven for 15 to 20 minutes.

5. Serve at once by setting each *papillote* on a plate.

4 tablespoons crème fraîche

8 red mullet fillets, about 2 ounces each

4 teaspoons sliced shallots

8 slices of lime

Salt and freshly ground pepper

N.B. YOU CAN USE SOLE OR SNAPPER INSTEAD OF RED MULLET.

. . . .

BARBECUED DUCK WITH PEACHES

Serves 4

1. Prepare the barbecue or preheat the broiler.

2. Mix the honey, 1/4 cup water, and lemon juice over medium heat and stir until dissolved. This step will take a couple of minutes. Let cool for 5 minutes.

2 duck *magrets* (breasts)

1 teaspoon honey

Juice of 1/2 lemon

INGREDIENTS

¹/₂ teaspoon butter

4 yellow peaches or nectarines, pitted and cut into slices (8 per peach)

Salt and freshly ground pepper

3. Pour half of the honey mixture on the duck breasts.

4. Melt the butter in a skillet over medium heat and add the peach slices. Pour the rest of the honey mixture over and cook for a few minutes until the peaches are tender but not mushy.

5. Grill the duck *magrets* 3 minutes on each side. Let rest a few minutes, and slice on the bias. Plate and cover with the peaches and their juice.

N.B. SERVING THIS DISH WITH A GREEN VEGETABLE LIKE ZUCCHINI OR HARICOTS VERTS ADDS COLOR AND TAKES CARE OF YOUR VEGGIES PORTION.

. . . .

CHICKEN WITH PASTIS

Serves 8

Pastis: the Provençal drink par excellence.

Let me be honest: I have never been able to drink pastis, the anise-based liquor . . . too strong for me. Many of my women friends feel the same. One can get drunk fast. I love the smell of it, but when I grew up, I saw too many village pétanque *players drinking lots of pastis, and the final picture was not so nice. It goes to your head pretty quickly, and the stuff being so refreshing (an ounce or so mixed with water and ice), it's easy to go for seconds and thirds.*

Now, there is finally an alternative, and I must say I love it. It's pastis without the alcohol and without the sugar. On the other hand, to cook with pastis you must use the real thing, and it is delicious and available in wine stores.

In Provence, we cook rabbit with it, and my friend Georgette introduced me to this dish years ago. I've tried it with chicken for my New York friends and find the dish equally yummy. One more way to cook chicken. All my friends love it.

1. Mix the pastis and oil. Season with salt and pepper to taste.

2. Arrange the chicken pieces in one layer in a shallow dish. Drizzle with the marinade and cover the dish with plastic. Refrigerate for 2 hours (it's even better to do the day before and let marinate overnight).

3. Warm the 3 tablespoons of oil in a *cocotte* over medium heat. Add the onions and cook until softened, about 6 minutes. Add the tomatoes, garlic, and fennel seeds. Continue cooking for 15 minutes, stirring occasionally.

4. Add the chicken pieces and the marinade to the *cocotte*. Cover and simmer over medium-low heat for about 30 minutes. Add the olives and 1/3 of the basil. Cover and continue cooking until the chicken is tender, about 30 minutes. Season with salt and pepper to taste and garnish with the rest of the basil. Serve immediately.

INGREDIENTS

FOR THE MARINADE:

2/3 cup pastis

1/3 cup olive oil

Salt and freshly ground pepper

1 3-pound chicken cut into 8 pieces

3 tablespoons olive oil

2 onions, peeled and sliced

4 tomatoes, diced

4 cloves garlic, minced

2 teaspoons fennel seeds

2/3 cup black olives, pitted and chopped

1 cup basil, slivered

Salt and freshly ground pepper

N.B. YOU CAN SERVE THIS WITH RICE OR NOODLES AND DRINK A RED CÔTES DU RHÔNE.

TRICOLOR PEPPERS

Serves 4

Peppers are another New World plant that has taken root in a big way in the Old. Far more than with asparagus, color counts for peppers' taste. The common green variety, really only a pepper picked unripe, is less subtle and less delicately flavored. The reds and yellows, which appear later, have had more of a chance to soak up the sun, making their skin thinner and more tender and their flesh sweeter. These baubles dazzle the eye and palate alike. They can be enjoyed equally well raw in a salad or stewed or grilled to enhance their extraordinary sweetness. As with strawberries, small ugly specimens are better than airbrushed symmetrical giants.

I love the taste and the color and the versatility of this yummy vegetable, but I must confess that I don't understand people who spend the time roasting them to get rid of the skin. I love the skin, which has lots of nutrients I want to keep. Almost every Saturday I buy one or two of each color at the market, and here is one way I consume them.

INGREDIENTS

6 sweet peppers (2 each of red, orange, yellow)

1. Cut the peppers in half through the stem. Discard the stems, ribs, and seeds. Cut into large strips.

2. Put the red peppers at the bottom of a steamer, followed by the orange and yellow. Steam for 6 to 8 minutes. Voilà.

I serve them hot as a side dish with fish, white meat, or pasta dishes. All one needs to add is a drizzle of olive oil and a dash of seasoning. I refrigerate the leftovers, then use them for lunch during the week, with a piece of leftover chicken, tuna, or salmon; or a few shrimp; or for a salad lunch over some mixed greens and a hard-boiled egg or chunks of feta cheese. Then I add a mustard-vinegar-oil dressing and always lots of chopped parsley. And, of course, the simplest thing is to serve them at room temperature on a *tartine* (a thick slice of country or sourdough bread) with a few grains of salt, a drizzle of olive oil, and parsley.

WATERCRESS COULIS

Serves 4

1. Rinse the watercress well, and steam for 5 minutes.

2. Toss with the crème fraîche (or equivalent). Toss with the egg yolks and nutmeg, and season with salt and pepper to taste. Serve immediately.

INGREDIENTS

2 bunches watercress

4 tablespoons crème fraîche, sour cream, or yogurt

2 egg yolks

1/4 teaspoon freshly grated nutmeg

Salt and freshly ground pepper

EGGPLANT TAPENADE

Serves 4

2 medium eggplants,
unpeeled, cut into 1-inch-
thick slices

4 tablespoons olive oil

1 red onion, peeled and
thinly sliced

2 cups chopped tomatoes

½ cup red wine vinegar

2 tablespoons capers

8 pitted green olives

8 pitted black olives

Salt and freshly ground
pepper

1. Salt the eggplant slices, and let stand for 20 minutes. Rinse with cold water, and pat dry. (This process makes the eggplant more tender and less bitter.)

2. Warm the oil over medium heat. Cook the eggplant and onion until brown and lightly crisp. Remove from the pan.

3. Add the tomatoes and vinegar to the pan, and cook for a few minutes over medium heat. Add the capers and olives, and season with salt and pepper to taste. Toss with the eggplant and onion, and serve immediately.

. . . .

VEGETABLES WITH YOGURT DRESSING

Serves 6

2 teaspoons Meaux
mustard

2 tablespoons red wine
vinegar

6 tablespoons walnut or
hazelnut oil

½ cup yogurt

1. Put the mustard and vinegar in a bowl, and mix well. Whisk in the oil, then add the yogurt and chives. Season with salt and pepper to taste. Whisk well.

2. Pour the dressing over the remaining ingredients, and toss gently. Serve with pita bread.

INGREDIENTS

2 tablespoons chopped chives

Salt and freshly ground pepper

6 medium new potatoes, peeled and sliced, and cooked in boiling water for 10 minutes

1 large cucumber, peeled and cubed

2 tomatoes, cut into 8 pieces

4 celery stalks, cut into ½-inch pieces

½ cup raisins

. . . .

VIVA LA PLANCHA

Barbecue, as I've said, is our secret weapon in summer. Few French people will admit it, but they envy the American—and Australian—knack for the grill, with its *Quest for Fire* immediacy to food. In the past few decades I've seen many of my compatriots return from visits to America toting barbecue paraphernalia.

Barbecue is not only perfect for entertaining. It also fits in with the trend among many French to desacralize gastronomy, keeping what is pure and elemental while forgoing the stuffiness of service and dining ritual—women still bring their lapdogs to restaurants, but men wear ties less often. Some formalities will persist, as they should: close though the French may get to a BBQ shack, you will never find an eatery serving a precious Salers steak, from four-year-old Auvergne cows, on paper plates. And ketchup on fries? *Jamais.* But in most other respects, the French have shown themselves eager adaptors of this excellent American ritual. At Houston's renowned Goode Company Barbeque, I observed a sign inviting patrons to bring their own meat in for barbecuing—there, deep in the heart of Texas, an invitation to planned and thoughtful eating that could warm even a French woman's heart. Nowadays in France—all over Europe, really—you can buy any model Weber barbecue you want, including gas grills like the one we've enjoyed in New York for sixteen years!

I fell in love with barbecue the first time Edward grilled me a steak. A friend had given us an extraordinary bottle of red wine, and so Edward decided to splurge on a porterhouse. As the grill heated he sprinkled the meat with just a few small pieces of garlic here and there and poured on the juice of a lemon, then grilled it with some portobello mushrooms. Seasoning took place at the table. Of such simple things are memories made.

The French being the French, and perpetually innovating in their obsessions with food, quality, and pleasure, they have taken a turn back to the future, rediscovering a nineteenth-century Spanish invention that does the grill one better, at least healthwise. *La plancha,* a magically conductive steel griddle, allows one to cook very fast without much fat, and because it is a flat, unbroken surface, there is less risk of charring the food. Purists will complain that this defeats the purpose of barbecue, but doctors agree that charred food can be carcinogenic—don't we have enough of that in our food chain already?

Though it wants for the glow of coals, the *plancha* offers the great virtue of cooking, as chefs say, *à la minute*—basically, just before you're sitting down to eat. At the same time it preserves the textures and flavors of fresh produce. And not least, it can be used both indoors and out. The Spanish have used the *plancha* for years to make tapas, their very extemporaneous and varied food of little servings, which, naturally, the French adore. Variety is no problem, because you can cook most things in a matter of minutes once the *plancha* is really hot.

Maybe it was my American nostalgia. Or maybe it was the odd pleasure of dislocation, as Woody Allen expresses it: "When I'm in Paris I want to be in New York, and when I am in New York I wish I were in Paris." But one year Edward and I were in Spain around Thanksgiving, and I longed for turkey. A friend in Barcelona indulged me with a delightful Spanish interpretation of turkey scaloppine with Marsala and sage. Just two hours before our expatriate version of the feast that would have taken all day to prepare *à l'américaine,* she had put a small slice of the incomparable Iberico ham on each turkey slice and overlaid that with a sliver of mozzarella and some fresh sage leaves. She then rolled up the scaloppines and secured each with toothpicks before transferring them to a deep dish; over it all she poured some Marsala (sherry works well, too), olive oil, and a dash of salt and pepper. After basting the scaloppines a few times, she popped them into the fridge until it was time to cook them: eight to ten minutes on the preheated *plancha.* In the last two minutes, she added the lovely accompaniment of apple slices. We enjoyed it with a wonderful Rioja, but I have served the meal at home very happily with a good Zinfandel. Anyone who has suffered the blandness of the comical misnomer that is Butterball should give this delicious Thanksgiving *à la catalan* a try. It may not supplant the traditional roast turkey with all the fixings in autumn, but in summer, you'll be thankful for an easy little taste of tradition while the leaves are still on the trees. The only thing missing will be the apples. Apples can be found in summer, as everything can, but they aren't meant to be. And with so many alternatives, we shouldn't miss them too much.

TUTTI FRUTTI

The summer offers such an orgy of fruits that I luxuriate in them *au naturel.* Not that *I'm* in the altogether; they are. I eat them as freshly picked as possible, at room temperature, usually as plain as nature gave them to us. (Okay, occasionally I put a dollop of vanilla ice cream on the berries or peaches.) Strawberries, blueberries, blackberries, varieties of cherries, white peaches, yellow peaches, plums large and small, apricots, figs, and all sorts of melons: most of the fruits you can name are summer fruits, and in summer they are so plentiful that even the big supermarkets sometimes have something good to offer. Typically, though, they overchill produce, and it sits past its prime. Fortunately, where there are fresh vegetables, there are also fresh fruits. And if you can't be bothered to seek them both out, you are depriving yourself of one of the most essential ways French women fill their summers with eating pleasure without getting fat. (You're also missing the convenience of a perfect dessert that needs virtually no preparation.)

True, French women have it a little easier than most, with a gastronomic culture built around the market and a government that subsidizes the quality, not the quantity, of its agriculture. But that's the way the people have always had it, and that's the way they want it. In America, as elsewhere, supply chases demand. A relative indifference to premium summer produce is precisely what limits its availability. But if you plant it, they will come. Farmers' markets are the future, at least concerning those foodstuffs in which freshness counts. If there isn't a market very near you now, chances are there will be soon. Meanwhile, vote with your feet and find the nearest one. Don't miss out. With a balanced consumption of fruit and a cultivated taste for its splendors, summer can be a season-long holiday from the risk of getting fat. And we all deserve that kind of a break today, don't we?

Even in an ideal world, not all the fruits of summer are destined to be eaten fresh, and the perfectly ripe cannot always be found. Sometimes we must make do with what we can find, even in farmers' markets. Apricots are one of my very favorite fruits, but as motivated as I am, I'm still hard pressed to find great ones, save right off the tree. More often than not, most of what's for sale tends to be woolly and lacking in that true apricot flavor, knowledge of which more often comes from preserves than from encounters with ripe apricots. Cooked preparations concentrate the flavors and the natural sugars. Those of you who have experienced a fresh, juicy apricot can vouch for the rarity of same at any distance from where the best grow—in Turkey or California, for example. In my part of Provence they cultivate an *acidulée* variety available for only a few weeks. That doesn't give one much time. We savor what we can. At home, my mother would preserve them, to produce wonderful tarts in the winter. (Sour cherries and rhubarb are other favorites of the women in my family, who tend to like their sweetness cut with a bit of tartness.)

BAKED APRICOTS

Serves 4

INGREDIENTS

16 apricots, halved and pitted
1 teaspoon vanilla
6 ounces dry vermouth
3 ounces honey

1. Preheat the oven to 350 degrees.

2. Lay the apricots skin-side up in overlapping rows in an ovenproof dish. Mix the vanilla with the vermouth, and pour over the apricots. Drizzle the honey over, and bake in the preheated oven for 20 minutes, until the apricots are tender.

3. Allow to cool, then chill. Serve with crème fraîche or whipped cream (on top of yogurt is another option).

· ·

GRILLED PEACHES WITH CINNAMON AND ROSEMARY

Serves 4

Peaches, like apricots, demand to be eaten when perfectly ripe, but because they bruise so easily, they are frequently picked when they feel like baseballs. Set aside, they will mature, but you can't expect the peachiness of a ripe picking. Keep an eye out for those—you'll know them by the scent. Lesser peaches can be grilled, however, with excellent results.

1. Preheat the broiler if you plan to use it instead of the grill.

2. Rinse the peaches, pat dry, cut in half, and remove the pits. Place the peach halves in a baking dish. Mix the sugar and cinnamon, stir in the oil, and brush the mixture over the peaches. Sprinkle with the rosemary. Marinate for 10 minutes, turning over and basting once.

3. Broil or grill the marinated peaches for 2 to 3 minutes on each side, until they are tender but not soft. Serve immediately, alone or with a scoop of vanilla or cinnamon ice cream.

INGREDIENTS

4 peaches

1 tablespoon sugar

⅛ teaspoon cinnamon

2 tablespoons canola oil

4 sprigs rosemary, minced

FIGS WITH RICOTTA

Serves 4

INGREDIENTS

4 tablespoons honey
1 tablespoon orange zest
4 strips orange peel
8 fresh figs
1 cup ricotta cheese

1. Mix ½ cup water, honey, zest, and orange strips in a large skillet over medium heat, stirring until the honey has dissolved, about 2 minutes. Bring to a boil, and cook until the syrup has reduced and thickened, 5 minutes or so.

2. Remove from the heat. Add the figs to the pan, and gently coat with the syrup.

3. Spoon ¼ cup ricotta into each serving bowl, add two figs, and drizzle with syrup.

. . . .

BRINGING SUMMER INDOORS

The indoor gardener can do herself a favor with potted herbs. Among them, terribly delicate basil almost never makes it to market with its leaves intact; a small potted plant set on a windowsill will repay the small effort of its cultivation with fragrant leaves. As for other types of indoor planting, they're almost beside the point, since summer is to be met on its own turf, strictly outside. You hardly need visit a botanical garden, though I love doing that, to see the seasonal handiwork. The trees may have lost their blossoms, but the roses are out, and so are all the annuals—among my personal favorites, salvia, lantana, and cosmos.

The feast is not so moveable for the seasonal container gardener, as a lot of outdoor plants simply don't do well indoors. Geraniums, for example, thrive in our terrace pots and window boxes but are far from happy to come inside. The potted plants that can make the migration well enough are the delicate ones, such as miniature roses and even marigolds, which as always can be complemented with *plantes vertes* for bulk and contrast, although their life span inside is akin to those of cut flowers. If you are lucky enough to have watched your garden grow, fresh-cut flowers are your reward. In her flower shop my acquaintance Anaïs has a sign reading *"Qui plante son jardin plante son bonheur"*—she who plants her garden plants her happiness—and I couldn't put it better. For the rest of us there is the surrogate garden of the greenmarket or the florist.

But even with flowers in summer, abundance has its limitations. I certainly never saw impatiens while I was growing up in France or when I first came to America, but after 1990 they were ubiquitous. Fed by watering systems and adopted as "a look" by international hotel and resort chains, impatiens can be seen from Florida to the Middle East, from China to Europe, and even on our terrace before we'd had enough of them. They are hardy, impatient to bloom, and provide a nice blanket of color, especially in shady areas; but they have simply become too commonplace. Even in the season of abundance, more than enough can spoil a good thing.

• A Week's Menu for Summer •

Breakfast

Blueberry Baby Smoothie
(www.mireilleguiliano
.com)
1 slice multigrain bread,
toasted and buttered
1-ounce slice boiled ham
Coffee or tea

Lunch

Vichyssoise (page 117)
1 hard-boiled egg
1 slice watermelon
Noncaloric beverage

Dinner

Grilled chicken with thyme
Eggplant Tapenade
(page 128)
1 ear of corn on the cob
Green salad
1 serving Grilled Peaches
with Cinnamon and
Rosemary (page 135)
1 glass white, rosé, or red
wine

Breakfast

1 ounce Jarlsberg cheese
½ cup muesli
½ cup milk
½ cup strawberries
Coffee or tea

Lunch

Tomato-mozzarella salad
1 slice country bread
1 cup cherries
Noncaloric beverage

Dinner

Snapper with Almonds
(www.mireilleguiliano
.com)
3 ounces asparagus with
1 teaspoon olive oil
½ cup potatoes
Mireille's Simple Tomato
Salad (page 120)
1 cup mixed fruit salad
1 glass rosé or red wine

• A Week's Menu for Summer •

WEDNESDAY

Breakfast

2 prunes
1 soft-boiled egg
1-ounce slice of salami or
    saucisson
2 slices baguette, buttered
Coffee or tea

Lunch

Cold Beet and Yogurt
    Summer Soup
    (www.mireilleguiliano
    .com)
3 ounces fish
1/2 cup yogurt
1 slice olive bread
1 nectarine
Noncaloric beverage

Dinner

Orecchiette with Tuna and
    Zucchini (page 122)
Green salad
1 slice melon
1 glass red wine

THURSDAY

Breakfast

1 slice prosciutto
1/2 cup bran cereal
1/2 cup milk
1/2 cup raspberries
Coffee or tea

Lunch

Yogurt with cucumber
1/2 cup green vegetables
3 fresh apricots
Noncaloric beverage

Dinner

4 ounces veal scaloppine
1 large grilled tomato
2/3 cup Brown Rice with Peas
    (page 45)
1 cup mixed berries
1 glass white or red wine

• A Week's Menu for Summer •

<table>
<tr><td>

Breakfast

½ cup tomato juice
½ cup yogurt
1 cup mixed berries
1 slice whole wheat bread,
    toasted and buttered
Coffee or tea

Lunch

Ratatouille
    (www.mireilleguiliano
    .com)
1 slice country bread
1 ounce goat cheese
1 peach
1 square chocolate
Noncaloric beverage

Dinner

Halibut *en Papillote*
    (www.mireilleguiliano
    .com)
Watercress Coulis (page 127)
1 teaspoon unsalted butter
1 ounce blue cheese
3 crackers
2 plums
1 glass white or red wine

</td><td>

Breakfast

½ cup freshly squeezed
    orange juice or 1 orange
½ cup yogurt
1 *pain au chocolat* or 1 slice
    raisin bread
Coffee or tea

Lunch

Melon Soup (page 116)
Mini cheese tray (3 types,
    1 ounce each)
1 slice peasant bread
Green salad
1 bowl strawberries
Noncaloric beverage

Dinner

Red Mullet with Spinach *en
    Papillote* (page 122)
½ cup Tricolor Peppers
    (page 126)
Mesclun salad
1 slice blueberry tart
1 glass Champagne or
    sparkling wine or white
    wine

</td></tr>
</table>

• A Week's Menu for Summer •

SUNDAY

Breakfast

½ cup mixed berries
½ cup yogurt
1 croissant
Coffee or tea

Lunch

Grilled Steak with Wine
    Sauce (page 167)
Grilled vegetables
Green salad
1 cup strawberries with
    a scoop of vanilla ice
    cream
1 glass red wine

Dinner

1 bowl cold soup (such as
    beet, page 113, or
    fennel, page 114)
1 slice country bread
Salad with olives and hard-
    boiled egg
2 yellow plums

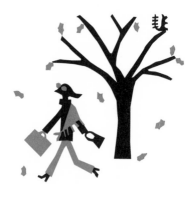

4

For many of us, no season's passing is mourned as summer's is. We manage every time not to notice how easy our lives have become in summer. We often complain that it's not what it used to be, more like the rest of our busy year. But even those who work right through the season (as most now do) can't deny the attitude of relative laissez-faire: the pace is slackened, the energy dampened a bit, by the routine absence of colleagues in any given week. People work with a weekend-to-weekend mentality.

We don't appreciate the relative ease until everyone snaps back to attention. The first Monday in September is Labor Day, when everyone squeezes in one more weekend of vacation, mental or otherwise. The Going Back to School sales season and drama end for us. The curtain goes up on a new academic year . . . the games begin. In my business, as in many, fall is the big selling season. Once again people are watching and begin keeping score.

This can be a rude awakening. While basking in summer, we tend not to address the big strategic issues such as unfulfilled professional or emotional hopes. But a fresh start can be quite energizing, too. Taking up new challenges, dealing more purposefully with work and goals: it can all add up to real stimulation, with genuine psychic and financial rewards. But also stress. There are only so many waking hours in a day. As we return to multitasking full speed, we may be psyched overall, but we also tend to lose focus on ourselves and, in a broader sense, on our place in nature. With everyone expecting more from us and holiday travel—worse yet: holiday travelers!—soon to descend on us, our equilibrium can get swamped. And sometimes we get fat. We are not alone in this: many other mammals start layering it on as the chill permeates the air—though admittedly they stop eating almost entirely in the months thereafter. (Compensations.) But what are we humans to do? *C'est la vie, non?*

It's true that nature and tradition have ordained autumn as the last stop on summer's free ride of on-demand bounty, of peak flavor with relatively few calories. But the season is glorious in its own way: "Thou hast thy music too," as Keats wrote, addressing autumn's inferiority complex compared with spring. I would not trade for anything the rustle of fall leaves, much less the changing light and hues of the landscape, the first smell of a neighbor's fire. When I first arrived in Weston, Massachusetts, as an exchange student, it was fall, and I had not yet grown round. Being in New England, home of the Pilgrims, I could not have felt a more intense sense of arriving in America. It was then that I first celebrated Thanksgiving, the American holiday par excellence. I still remember my first taste of cranberry dressing, my first tumble in a pile of leaves of American oak and maple. There was no better place to observe the change of colors, and I became hooked on that seasonal rite. Today it can breed some anxiety among the New Englanders overrun with us gawkers, and I have even noticed people stressing out over missing the peak weekend when the leaves "turn"—such is the modern condition! At the time, though, foliage was a joyous discovery.

But nature never intended this time to be frittered away in chasing the leaves. In fact, our modern rite of back-to-school, back-to-work is perfectly consistent with nature's plan, although in a different guise. This has always been the time to reap—in fact, for most of history, to reap for your life! Not so long ago, there was no surviving the winter without an abundance of those fruits of the earth that could be laid in for the mostly lifeless months ahead. (In the wine business, too, a bad harvest is death, at least in retail terms.)

I suppose one positive effect of mass agribusiness is to have freed those of us in the developed world from the fear of starvation. Perpetual plenitude, however, comes at a price: an impaired sense of seasonal rhythm and of pacing ourselves. Unlike summer, autumn doesn't give us irresistible guidance regarding how to eat. Our exertions also tend to become more sedentary. Still, there are meaningful ways of registering the season in our minds and bodies. You don't have to thresh your own wheat, but you can do better than collecting a couple of decorative gourds.

If you prefer taking your color cues from the landscape rather than from Paris, Milan, or New York, try to look beyond the leaf pile embedded in our cultural consciousness. Even where the colors never change, children in autumn are made to draw leaves. True, the leaves are the season's glory, and outdoor flowers don't beckon to us as they do in spring and summer. But many do last well past summer, and the season "set[s] budding more / And still more, later flowers for the bees" (Keats *encore*)—else there would be no honey to harvest. Our favorite late bloomer is the chrysanthemum. Mums have become widely available in plastic containers, which we place inside decorative pots, often accented with ivy or maidengrass.

Now, with so many colors of mums as well as varieties, from pompon to spider, there's much one can do with size, shape, and color; but for my taste, less is *toujours* more, and two colors are quite enough. The plants are inexpensive enough that you can buy a lot, but consider the setting: one might call out for one or two plants, another for a dozen. Whether you are going for something spare or florabundant, don't dilute the effect with a little of this and a little of that— stick with one type. Depending on the weather and the state of our plants, we might start early with mums, refreshing with new plants late in the season.

Other flowers we enjoy early and late into fall are daisies, especially the perennial golden *Rudbeckia*, or black-eyed Susan. These also come in pots, but they don't do well indoors, so we enjoy them on the terrace for as long as they last. We have some six-inch pots of tiny asters that work indoors or out, and we bring them in, placing them in corners where they don't rival the mums, a defiant splash of color and life.

In fall we really have to begin to carve out our personal time and relaxation or we run the risk of not having any. Some call this deprivation virtue, but I call it a recipe for overeating. It shouldn't take much rousing to go out for a good long walk in fall, especially in a park. In New York and Paris I love the energy on the streets when everyone is back from *les congés d'été*—the summer holidays. I enjoy meeting a friend or a relative (one I like) for brunch. We might then take a stroll through a new museum exhibition or (less edifying, perhaps) through SoHo's stores—each in its way a wonderful distraction for a fall weekend. But make the plan and stick with it. Relentless self-application may seem ambitious, but it takes the edge off your A game. Successful people know how to let it alone.

Fall is also a good time to reacquaint yourself with moderate free weights, especially if you're over forty. A bit of extremely simple resistance training is a French woman's answer to the hours of working aerobic machines that many American women favor. The French author Colette, with her proto-Pilates contraptions, was the first modern woman to work out. As I've said, short but focused intervals of exertion several times a week are all you need to be physically healthy. (The rest we do for our head.) A little goes a long way, so don't let extremism overtake you. In the end, those who know how to stay fit while enjoying life come out ahead, mentally and physically.

Overall, a key to managing the uptick of seasonal stress is to increase your physical exertion indoors. Let's face it, the shorter the days, the less time you'll spend outside, where there is no couch or flat screen. I walk and cycle as much as I can. And take the stairs. But I also turn more regularly to yoga. I do more work around the house as well. Sometimes we must make do with a short interior journey, such as focusing on a simple task—the French woman's zen. The smallest oases of serenity placed throughout the day can make all the difference to your heart and mental health.

Speaking of short journeys, my grandmother devised the perfect outdoor one for early Sunday mornings in the fall. We'd walk into the forest, where, under the canopy of trees not yet denuded, the light would dance all around us as we stood in the utter silence, drinking in all the wonderful odors of decay from the humid *sous-bois* (forest floor), a bit like tasting an old wine. (There is, incidentally, a specifically autumnal gastronomy connected with the business of decay. The noble rot on grapes gives some wines their excellence; a magnificent Stilton could be mistaken for another cheese left out too long. There's sometimes a fine line between perfection and ruin.)

In the wood, we would catch sight of the occasional deer that hadn't caught a whiff of us. Or we would collect mushrooms, guided by my grandmother's faultless eye for distinguishing what was delicious from what was lethal in this dappled other world just a few hundred meters from her garden. A far cry from the supermarket shrink-wrapped buttons that may not kill you, but the taste is about equal to the thrill of finding them. But even more salutary was being out there in perfect stillness, in another world.

Nature is full of marvelous microcosms we can enter,

even if only mentally. Another of these was the world of my father's beehives.

Honey's dark gold reminds me of fall. And inevitably it reminds me of first learning to gather the bees' bounty. While we can keep and eat honey all year round (see how I use it in various recipes throughout the seasons), we harvest it in late spring and finally in late fall, when "the maturing sun" conspires with the season

> *to set budding more,*
> *And still more, later flowers for the bees,*
> *Until they think warm days will never cease,*
> *For Summer has o'er-brimm'd their clammy cells.*

Just what those insects were up to in those "clammy cells" to produce such a heavenly food was a mystery. As an eight-year-old I couldn't quite fathom that bees collect the nectar from flowers and transform it in their honey stomachs. The *apiculteur* (beekeeper) loved to explain this to me over and over, and I never tired of hearing the story. The bees were his third hobby, the other two being his garden and his pigeons.

Granted the beekeeper was only an amateur, but my father seemed to know everything about keeping the colony clean, the queen healthy, and her subjects working—all conditions vital to a good harvest. Somewhat to my mother's annoyance, he kept a few hives square in the middle of the flower gardens. In bee real estate, location really is everything. We watched with great fascination, though Father was not particularly good at finding age-appropriate terms to explain how the queen was the only sexually developed female in the hive, how she mates with all the stout male bees, receiving millions of anonymous sperm cells and laying up to three thousand eggs in one day. Hard to imagine how the birds and the bees (or the bees, at least) ever became delicate models of sex education. The queen is a father's nightmare. Anyway, the game was more show than tell, and we spent hours and hours following the bees as witness to their purposeful busyness.

A solemn if scary moment was when I'd be allowed to put on long gloves and a straw hat with a veil of netting to help my father tend the apiary. There was no more exciting event than the early fall extraction of the honeycomb from the hive. As a child I felt a certain poignancy in seeing the fruit of my little friends' ceaseless labors taken from them. But the bees seemed to trust my father, and they were not wrong. Of course he knew when the honey was ripe for harvest, and exactly how much to leave them so the colony could survive the cold months without flowers. He said they made more than enough for themselves, and so we were welcome to the rest.

Everyone loved the honey, but only my father and I loved the comb. It was, first of all, beautiful to look at, a gorgeous waxen lattice of painstaking construction, an insect Chartres cathedral. It was also the choice of honey connoisseurs. We cut it up and ate it like a house of gingerbread, finally forgetting the life-and-death struggle of the bees to make it. Sometimes I'd mix it with my favorite cheese, *petit Suisse,* although today I would substitute homemade yogurt. The rest of the harvest remained liquid honey, poured into jars, and consumed in countless ways during the year or given away as gifts.

In winter, when on occasion breakfast was a thick slice of

bread with a thick slice of butter drizzled with honey, we would always feel thankful for our father's rapprochement with the bees, even without knowing what is known today: that honey, in particular darker varieties, is a significant source of antioxidants. It also had uses in ancient Egyptian and Vedic medicine and, until the development of antibiotics, was used to inhibit bacterial growth and heal wounds. It still makes a good facial toner. There is also a very simple reason French women keep honey in their diet: because it's so sweet (approximately one and a half times as sweet as white sugar), as well as divinely flavorful, you can use less—in my case, about half the amount of processed sugar. It's also more slowly digested, therefore less likely to cause the unpleasant effects of blood-glucose spikes. And with honey, you'll never want for variety: there are about three hundred kinds. My preferences: acacia, clover, brambles, and lavender. You can taste the flowers of summer in the honey of fall. Don't worry if it appears cloudy; it stays edible for years—bacteria may spoil other foods but not the taste of honey.

Sometimes I add a few drops of honey to the water I sip during long walks or other exercise. When cooking or baking, I substitute half the sugar in a recipe with honey. I drizzle it over thick plain yogurt, waffles, or pancakes. And my New York friends adore receiving honey from Provence. In fairness, I should point out that my Provence friends love to receive the fabulous maple syrup from my adoptive homeland. This New World sugar substitute, popularized in the colonies when sugar was heavily taxed, also boasts health benefits, including concentrations of essential minerals such as manganese, to say nothing of its own distinctive earthy flavors.

Some stereotypes are true: Italians eat pasta, Asians eat rice, and the French eat potatoes. In fact, these were cultural staples long before stereotypes existed. But one stereotype à la Atkins that has done harm is that of the potato as bad or junk food, starchy throwaway calories. The potato is actually filled with nutrients, and if we would speak of calories, a six-ounce potato has only a fourth of those in an equal portion of rice or pasta. *Vive la pomme de terre!* Oh, and did I mention vitamins? The potato has practically all of them, with a particular richness in C and the B gamut. And it is the most versatile vegetable: it marries well with anything. It becomes an offender only when deep-fried or when commandeered as a sour-cream-and-Cheddar delivery system.

When I was growing up, we ate potatoes in some shape or form at lunch—as one of the two vegetable accompaniments to fish or meat—an average of five days a week. The variations prevented any sense of spud monotony. There were steamed, roasted, or oven baked; mashed potatoes, potato salad, or, yes, even *frites* (though in careful moderation as a Sunday lunch treat). Different preparations called for different varieties: for example, we would never use new potatoes in the mash—not enough starch—though they roasted deliciously with rosemary or thyme. And some were precious: the famous and incomparable Noirmoutier, available only three months of the year, was as delicate, sweet, and (alas) pricey as potatoes get. A little steaming is all they require. On the other end of the spectrum, the common Idaho stands up well to baking, the Yukon Gold can take the deep-fry. À propos of deep-frying, a word of advice about so-called french fries: much of the problem is America's addiction to oil—the bad kind. If it is changed every twenty thousand miles and it's a trans fat (as is true in most fast-food restaurants), even one fry is too many. Ditto for those homemade ones steeped in Crisco, which if I were president would be a banned substance. If you have french fries at a good restaurant or make them yourself with a good fat, go ahead. Just remember that one Mont Blanc–sized serving you get in most dining establishments can feed the whole table.

POTATO GRATIN À LA NORMANDE

Serves 4

Normandy being apple and cheese country, lots of regional recipes include these two delicious staples. If you've never savored a perfectly ripe Pont l'Évêque (named for the town where it comes from in Calvados land), a soft cheese with a savory smell and a pronounced tang, you should try it. This recipe comes from a friend, and I especially like it for marrying protein with fruit flavor—a nice autumn lunch.

INGREDIENTS

18 ounces potatoes (russet or Idaho), peeled and sliced thinly

1 ounce walnuts, chopped

2 tablespoons unsalted butter

1. Preheat the oven to 375 degrees.

2. Cook the potatoes in slightly salted boiling water for 8 minutes, then drain.

3. While the potatoes cook, warm a nonstick frying pan, and toast the walnuts for a minute or two over medium heat. When cool, crumble and reserve.

4. Melt the butter in a frying pan over medium heat, add the apples, and let brown for 3 to 4 minutes while stirring. Cut the crust off the cheese, and slice the cheese thinly.

5. Butter a rectangular baking dish, and cover it with a layer of potatoes, then a layer of apples, a layer of cheese, and a sprinkle of walnuts. Continue layering until all the ingredients have been used. Top with sour cream, season with salt and pepper to taste, and bake in the preheated oven for 30 minutes.

INGREDIENTS

3 Granny Smith apples, peeled, cored, and cut into 8 pieces each

1 Pont l'Évêque cheese

7 ounces sour cream or crème fraîche

Salt and freshly ground pepper

N.B. A SIMPLE GREEN SALAD IS A PERFECT ACCOMPANIMENT TO THIS DISH, WHICH IS ALSO VERY GOOD SERVED WITH CHICKEN OR ANY WHITE MEAT.

MASHED POTATOES (*MAMIE'S* VERSION)
Serves 4

There is much dogma concerning great mashed potatoes. Some famous chefs regard it as essential to have almost equal parts potatoes and butter, but they would have been fired from my mother's kitchen: her customers expected butter when we ordered butter and potatoes when we were served potatoes. In other words, don't overdo the added fat. But do consider texture: it's very important to put the cooked potatoes while hot through a real vegetable mill or a potato ricer (a Cuisinart or blender will give you not a mash but a purée—by my taste buds, that's good only for wallpaper paste). Always add very hot milk first, then add the butter. For variety, you can replace the butter with olive oil (though it should be heated slightly and added at the end). You can also omit the milk by cooking the potatoes unpeeled and using the starchy water to wet the mash. Season with nutmeg, cumin, or curry, adding parsley, tarragon, dill, or basil. Another bit of dogma that I reject outright is the categorical good of a heavy dose of garlic. Much as I love to cook with garlic, which is wonderful for you, it overwhelms the potato flavors. Let the potato be a potato.

INGREDIENTS

2 pounds potatoes (Yukon Gold, russet, or Idaho), peeled and cut into 2-inch pieces

Salt and freshly ground pepper

3 tablespoons unsalted butter

¾ cup scalded milk (milk that has been heated to the point where it is almost boiling; regular or 2 percent)

1. Put the potatoes in a saucepan, and cover them with cold water. Add 1 teaspoon salt. Bring to a boil, cover partially, and cook over medium-low heat until tender, about 20 minutes.

2. Drain the potatoes, and put through a vegetable mill or potato ricer. Add the milk and whisk in the butter, then season with salt and pepper to taste. Serve immediately.

N.B. IF YOU NEED TO PREPARE MASHED POTATOES IN ADVANCE FOR A DINNER PARTY, YOU CAN PUT THEM IN A GLASS BOWL COVERED WITH ALUMINUM FOIL AND SET ATOP OF A POT FILLED WITH A FEW INCHES OF SIMMERING WATER. THEY WILL KEEP AT LEAST THIRTY MINUTES WITHOUT DRYING OUT. *MAMIE* WOULD STORE LEFTOVERS IN THE FRIDGE AND TWO DAYS LATER MAKE PATTIES THAT SHE WOULD REHEAT IN A BIT OF OIL WITH SOME SAUTÉED SHALLOTS. SHE COOKED THE PATTIES UNTIL THEY WERE NICELY BROWN ON EACH SIDE AND SERVED THEM WITH A GOOD TABLESPOON OF FRESHLY MINCED PARSLEY—ANOTHER QUICK SIDE DISH.

· · · · · · · · · ·

EN AUTOMNE

COD WITH POTATO SALAD

Serves 4

1. Put the potatoes in a saucepan, and cover them with cold water. Add 1 teaspoon salt, bring to a boil, and cook until tender, about 20 minutes, then drain.

2. Sauté the bacon until crisp in a nonstick pan. Pat dry on a paper towel.

3. Prepare the salad dressing: mix the oil, vinegar, mustard, and shallots, and season lightly with salt and pepper.

4. Put the cod in a pan, cover with cold water, and bring to a boil. Cover the pan, turn off the heat, and leave the fish to poach for 6 minutes. Drain, crumble the fish coarsely, set aside on a warm plate, and cover with foil.

5. Put some potatoes on each dish, add some cod and bacon, drizzle with dressing, and serve immediately.

INGREDIENTS

1½ pounds potatoes (Yukon Gold, White Rose, or Long Island white), peeled and cut into 2-inch pieces

Salt and freshly ground pepper

4 slices bacon, cut into ¼-inch pieces

5 tablespoons olive oil

2 tablespoons sherry vinegar

1 teaspoon Meaux mustard

2 tablespoons minced shallots

16 ounces cod

POTATO-OLIVE RAGOUT

Serves 4

Another fruit that marries brilliantly with potato is the olive, of which so many varieties are available, even in America. They travel well, being easy to preserve, and lose nothing in transit.

INGREDIENTS

3 tablespoons olive oil

1 pound potatoes (fingerlings, small reds, ruby crescent, or a mixture), peeled and cut like big, fat french fries

1 orange or yellow pepper, seeds removed, julienned

1 red pepper, seeds removed, julienned

2 cloves garlic, peeled and minced

2 shallots, minced

2 lemons, washed and quartered

6 ounces green olives, pitted

Salt and freshly ground pepper

4 tablespoons coarsely chopped cilantro

1. Warm the oil in a large nonstick pan over high heat. Add the potatoes and brown on all sides. Add the peppers, garlic, shallots, and lemon, and sauté for a few minutes. Add the olives, season with salt and pepper to taste, and cover. Cook over low heat until the vegetables are tender, about 10 minutes.

2. Add the cilantro, mix well, and serve immediately.

ULTRA RAPIDE MASHED YUKONS

Serves 4

1. Cut the washed but unpeeled potatoes into 1-inch chunks. Put in a medium saucepan with 1/2 teaspoon salt and enough water to cover. Bring to a boil, then lower the heat and simmer until tender, 10 to 15 minutes.

2. Drain the potatoes, and place them in 4 soup or cereal bowls. Mash roughly with a fork. To each bowl, season with ground coarse salt and pepper to taste, and drizzle on 1 teaspoon of the oil.

INGREDIENTS

1 1/2 pounds small Yukon Gold potatoes

Freshly ground coarse salt and pepper

4 teaspoons olive oil

. . . .

VEGETABLES

CAULIFLOWER GRATIN

Serves 4

1. Preheat the oven to 375 degrees.

2. Remove the leaves from the cauliflower, cut out the central stem, and break into florets. Wash in cold water, then steam for about 6 minutes. Put the florets in a baking dish.

3. In a bowl, combine the eggs, milk, cumin, garlic, and shallots. Pour the mixture over

INGREDIENTS

2 pounds cauliflower

4 eggs

3/4 cup regular milk

1/2 teaspoon ground cumin

2 cloves garlic, peeled and minced

2 shallots, minced

INGREDIENTS

Generous ½ cup fresh
bread crumbs

4 ounces white wine

Salt and freshly ground
pepper

the cauliflower, and sprinkle with bread crumbs. Add the wine to the baking dish, and bake in the preheated oven for 15 minutes. Season with salt and pepper to taste, and serve.

. . . .

ESCAROLE SAUTÉ

Serves 4

INGREDIENTS

2 pounds escarole

3 tablespoons olive oil

1 tablespoon minced shallot

Salt and freshly ground
pepper

1. Remove the tough outer leaves from the escarole. Wash thoroughly, and pat dry. Slice the leaves coarsely.

2. Warm the oil in a skillet over medium heat. Add the shallot, and cook until golden. Add the escarole, and cook over medium heat for 15 minutes, stirring occasionally, until tender. Season with salt and pepper to taste, and serve immediately.

. . . .

As the variety of vegetables bursting with natural flavor tapers off after summer, soups can tend to get a bit more complicated and hearty: people don't mind something a little heavier, and more things need to be added whereas one glorious flavor had sufficed before. Still, my favorite soups are the simplest. And fortunately, the fall greenmarkets are not completely depleted of delicious vegetables that don't need much help. There is a wealth of ripe peppers, and now the little chilies begin to appear, for those who like it hot. Parsnips can be made into a velvety base you'd swear was laden with cream. The soup that most says *fall* is squash, although the recipes work as well with either the last of the summer squash still coming in or the first of the winter squash just beginning to appear.

BUTTERSQUASH SOUP

Serves 4

1. Put the squash, onion, and potatoes in a large pot. Add the water. Bring to a boil, lower the heat, and cover. Simmer gently, stirring occasionally, for about 45 minutes.

2. Remove the vegetables with a slotted spoon, and purée in a food mill or food processor, using the cooking water to thin it out to the consistency desired. (If you're preparing soup ahead of time, use all the

INGREDIENTS

1 medium butternut squash, peeled and cut into large pieces

1 large yellow onion, peeled and coarsely chopped

½ pound red-skinned boiling potatoes (about 2 or 3), peeled and cut into ½-inch cubes

6 cups water

INGREDIENTS

4 tablespoons unsalted
butter

Salt and freshly ground
pepper

cooking water, since the soup will thicken as it stands.)

3. Just before serving, add to the heated soup the butter, and season with salt and pepper. Cook 2 minutes more, and serve.

N.B. JUST BEFORE SERVING, YOU CAN ADD FRESH PARSLEY FOR COLOR, OR 1/4 TEASPOON GRATED NUTMEG, OR BOTH. A SWIRL OF CRÈME FRAÎCHE OR SOUR CREAM WOULD BE NICE, TOO.

. . . .

LENTIL SOUP

Serves 4

INGREDIENTS

2 quarts vegetable stock

½ pound lentils

2 tablespoons olive oil

1 medium yellow onion,
peeled and chopped

1 clove garlic, peeled and
chopped

2 stalks celery, chopped

1 tablespoon chopped
parsley

1 14.5-ounce can diced
tomatoes

Salt and freshly ground
pepper

1. Bring the vegetable stock to a simmer, and drop in the lentils.

2. Heat the oil in a skillet, and add the onion, garlic, and celery. Cook until golden, 3 to 5 minutes. Add the parsley and tomatoes, and cook 8 to 10 minutes more.

3. After the lentils have been cooking for 35 to 40 minutes, add the onion mixture to pot and cover. Let simmer until the lentils are soft, 5 to 10 more minutes. Season with salt and pepper to taste, and serve immediately.

. . . .

FARFALLE WITH EDAMAME

Serves 4

Soybeans, a major harvest crop used for so many things, are something I discovered in America. Once the food of privation in Europe, today they are offered in Japanese restaurants as the amuse-bouche *edamame in their salted pods. You can also buy them shelled, fresh or frozen, and they make a good accompaniment to red meat—even pasta, as I learned from a young Asian woman selling them at the market. Curious at always seeing me buy them, she asked one day, "What do you do with them?" She revealed her own favorite way to enjoy them, and it has become one of mine.*

INGREDIENTS

1. Cook the farfalle in salted water according to package directions and stirring occasionally. In the last 5 minutes of cooking, add the edamame to the pot. Drain, reserving ⅓ cup of the pasta water.

2. Place the lemon zest and juice in a large pan over medium heat. Add the reserved pasta water, oil, and 2 ounces (½ cup) of the cheese. Mix well. Add the edamame and farfalle to the lemon mixture, and toss well to coat. Serve immediately, sprinkled with parsley and the remaining cheese. Season with pepper to taste.

12 ounces (4 cups) farfalle

Salt and freshly ground pepper

2 cups shelled edamame

Zest and juice of 1 lemon

2 tablespoons olive oil

3 ounces (about ¾ cup) grated Parmesan

2 tablespoons chopped parsley

MACARONI WITH SPINACH AND PANCETTA

Serves 4

INGREDIENTS

12 ounces (4 cups) macaroni, penne, or rigatoni

Salt and freshly ground pepper

1 tablespoon olive oil

3 ounces pancetta, diced into small pieces

½ cup dry white wine

1 pound spinach, washed

4 ounces (about 1 cup) grated Parmesan, or a mix of Parmesan and Pecorino

1. Cook the pasta in plenty of salted water, according to package directions and stirring occasionally.

2. Meanwhile, warm the oil in a large pan over low heat. Add the pancetta, and cook for 10 minutes. Add the white wine and spinach. Season with salt and pepper to taste, cover, and continue cooking over medium heat for 5 more minutes, until the spinach is wilted.

3. When the pasta is cooked, drain and add it to the pan with the pancetta and spinach. Add the cheese, and continue cooking for 5 minutes over medium heat, stirring continuously to mix the cheese with the pasta. Add some freshly ground pepper, and serve immediately.

CHICKEN AND HARICOTS VERTS SALAD

Serves 6

What Americans call string beans are known as French beans elsewhere, and haricots verts (green beans) are recognized as a slim variety of string beans. Before the nineteenth century the French didn't use them much because they were so expensive. Their wonderful color and snap have always made them seem like a token of springtime enjoyed in fall.

1. Bring 2 cups of water to a boil. Add the parsley, tarragon, bay leaf, onion, and salt. Drop the chicken into water, and poach for 12 minutes. Cool and cut the chicken into small pieces. (This step can be done in advance.)

2. For the dressing: Put the mustard and vinegar in a bowl, and mix well. Whisk in the oil, then add the cream and basil. Season with salt and pepper to taste.

3. Steam the beans for 8 minutes. Drain, and place in a bowl with the chicken, the dressing, and all the remaining ingredients, and toss gently.

INGREDIENTS

Sprig of parsley

Sprig of tarragon

1 bay leaf

½ an onion, peeled

Salt and freshly ground pepper

2 boneless, skinless chicken breasts

2 teaspoons Meaux mustard

2 tablespoons red wine vinegar

6 tablespoons olive oil

3 tablespoons heavy cream

2 tablespoons minced fresh basil

1 pound haricots verts

¾ pound mushrooms, cleaned and thinly sliced

1 cup Tricolor Peppers (page 126)

1 tablespoon lemon juice

1 cup coarsely chopped walnuts

SKATE WITH CAPERS

Serves 4

Skate is a wonderful fish; its thin, firm, but feathered white meat tastes sweet, with a surprisingly pleasant accent of ammonia. Because demand is low for this variety of ray, it is still very affordable in the United States. I had my first great skate dish in one of New York's top French restaurants some fifteen years ago and decided to look for it to cook at home. It's often available at the Union Square Greenmarket, and when I buy it, the next person in line inevitably asks, "How do you cook it?" My answer: "Pure and simple."

INGREDIENTS

1 tablespoon coarse salt

1 teaspoon crushed peppercorns

1 tablespoon red wine vinegar

4 skate wings (about 2 pounds)

2 tablespoons olive oil

4 tablespoons unsalted butter

2 medium tomatoes, cut in quarters

Juice of ½ lemon

4 tablespoons chopped parsley

¼ cup drained capers

1. Put 2 cups water in a large, deep skillet. Add the salt, peppercorns, and vinegar, and bring to a boil. Add the skate wings, and simmer for 8 minutes. (You may have to do two batches if your pan is not wide enough.) When poached, drain the fish, and set it aside on a warm plate. Cover with foil while preparing the sauce.

2. Warm the oil in a small saucepan, add the butter, and stir over medium heat until the butter is melted. Add the tomatoes, lemon juice, and 2 tablespoons parsley. Cook a few minutes, until the tomatoes soften. Add the capers, and cook another minute.

3. Put a skate wing on each plate. Top with the tomato-caper mixture, and sprinkle with the remaining parsley. You may also want to drizzle on a touch more oil. Serve with cauliflower gratin or mashed Yukon Gold potatoes.

MUSSELS IN WHITE WINE

Serves 4

A perfect dish to serve friends for a casual dinner. All you need to remember is to clean the mussels in advance. The best way is to scrub them with a small brush, then soak them in cold water with a teaspoon of salt for a couple of hours.

1. In a large pot, sauté the shallots in 1 tablespoon of the butter for 1 to 2 minutes. Add 1 tablespoon of the parsley, the thyme, white wine, and pepper to taste, and bring to a boil. Add the mussels, cover, and cook, shaking the pot once in a while, until the mussels open (it will take about 5 minutes). Discard any unopened mussels. Remove the remaining mussels to soup bowls.

2. Add the remaining butter to the pot. Stir until melted. Season with salt and pepper to taste. Pour the buttery juice over the mussels, and sprinkle with the remaining parsley. Serve with country bread to soak up any sauce, and have an empty bowl for collecting shells. Serve with the wine you used for cooking the mussels.

INGREDIENTS

2 tablespoons minced shallots

2 tablespoons unsalted butter

2 tablespoons minced parsley

1 sprig thyme

1 cup dry white wine

Salt and freshly ground pepper

4 pounds mussels, cleaned

TURKEY SCALOPPINE WITH PESTO

Serves 4

The French could pay more attention to turkey. Actually, Americans could, too: It's a bit of a shame that turkey tends to make only special guest appearances at the holidays, unless we buy it sliced in a deli sandwich. It's one of the leanest white meats, an excellent protein source, and it has become the base for my American version of veal scaloppine. My husband, who loves this dish, is always pleased when I announce a "green turkey night," signaling that with the turkey we will have a baked potato garnished with a dollop of pesto, as well as a portion of steamed broccoli. A turkey breast is much less a production to cook than a whole bird, and simpler still if you have the butcher slice it into scaloppine, as with a far more expensive breast of veal. I usually buy a fresh, organic turkey breast at Union Square Greenmarket, but they are easy to find. You can even order them on the Internet.

INGREDIENTS

FOR THE PESTO:

8 ounces fresh basil
½ cup pine nuts
2 cloves garlic, peeled
Pinch of salt
¾ to 1 cup olive oil
1 tablespoon grated
Parmesan cheese
1 tablespoon grated
Pecorino cheese

1. To make the pesto: Wash the basil, pat it dry, and place it in a mortar. Add the pine nuts, garlic, and salt. Pound the ingredients with a circular motion of the pestle until you obtain a green paste. Put the paste in a bowl, and add oil gradually. Add the cheeses just before serving, and more oil if necessary. (You can also do this in the food processor.) The pesto can be made in advance and frozen in small cubes for use when needed.

2. Warm 1 tablespoon oil in a frying pan over medium-high heat, and cook the turkey for a few minutes on each side. Add the

butter and lemon juice. Season with salt and pepper to taste. Add the pesto, and cook a few more minutes. If the sauce is on the dry side, add a few tablespoons of hot water. Mix well. Serve immediately.

FOR THE SCALOPPINE:

1 tablespoon olive oil

8 turkey scaloppines

½ tablespoon unsalted butter

Juice of ½ lemon

Salt and freshly ground pepper

N.B. MANY PEOPLE HAVE FAR TOO NARROW A NOTION OF PESTO. BASIL IS SUBLIME. I LOVE USING IT IN SUMMER WHEN IT FLOURISHES, AND I FREEZE PESTO MADE OF IT TO GET ME THROUGH THE REST OF THE YEAR. BUT DID YOU KNOW YOU CAN ALSO MAKE A ROSE-MARY PESTO? A HAZELNUT PESTO? FRENCH WOMEN DON'T HAVE IDÉES FIXES ABOUT SUCH THINGS AND LOVE TO INVENT THEIR OWN VARIATIONS. SO FEEL FREE. AUTUMN IS THE LAST CHANCE TO GET FRESH HERBS AT THE MARKET, SO NOW IS THE TIME TO MAKE PESTO.

GRILLED STEAK WITH WINE SAUCE

Serves 4

There is not much more a good steak needs than a bit of seasoning and grilling. While I don't generally recommend tampering with perfection, as the chilly months come on, we eventually put the Weber away. When we cook steak less primally, I love to use this wine sauce. It's perfectly natural that preparations become a little more elaborate as the season progresses. The richest ones are best had in winter. My friend and Alsatian compatriot Jean-Georges Vongerichten, chef and restaurateur known for the brilliant flavors, not the richness of his creations, used to make this dish when he apprenticed on the French Riviera at Louis Outhier's L'Oasis in La Napoule, a three-star restaurant of many nouvelle cuisine pilgrimages. I have adapted it slightly.

INGREDIENTS

1 cup plus 1 tablespoon red wine (separated), such as a Côtes du Rhône

2 cloves garlic, peeled and crushed

Salt and freshly ground pepper

1 tablespoon unsalted butter

2 16-ounce steaks

1. Combine 1 cup of the red wine and the garlic in a small saucepan. Bring to a boil over high heat, and reduce until syrupy (it will take about 10 minutes). Strain out the garlic, and season generously with salt and pepper. Return to low heat, and stir in the butter and the remaining tablespoon (uncooked) red wine.

2. Grill the steaks without adding anything to them. When ready, let them rest for a few minutes on a plate, then pour the sauce over them. Drink the rest of the wine with the meal.

. . . .

IF I COULD KEEP PEARS IN A BOTTLE

One of my most vivid memories of childhood is sitting on my grandmother's lap as she peeled pears and told me tales of her youth. Truth to tell, I also have a pretty vivid memory of licking the egg-and-cream batter from the bowl my Aunt Berthe had emptied (she was obligingly inefficient about getting it all out) for her Alsatian version of a tarte tatin, the classic upside-down apple pie. When the tart of apples or pears finally went into the oven, infusing the house with an incense of cinnamon and fruit, that was almost as good as the batter. It's said that nothing (except love of "mom") is as American as apple pie, yet for most the experience is only of the finished product, often a store-bought version. How many of us still enjoy waiting for it to come out of the oven, that same anticipation that was proverbially so unbearable for children that they would steal it from the window before it could cool? I love to imagine that sort of thing still happens, though it seems to be fading into myth, given our present lifestyle and relation to food.

Living in an area rich in apple and pear trees, my family had seemingly no end of recipes using them, as well as pleasures watching them grow. You could mark the weeks of the season as the tiny green fruit swelled, taking on the progressive colors of maturity until they were ready to be picked and stored in the *cagettes* (rectangular wooden crates). In the cool dark cellar, they would last all winter, losing only a bit of their crispness while growing sweeter.

Every year, my father would perform his impressive trick of putting a pear into a narrow-neck bottle. The bottle would then be filled with the highly alcoholic eau-de-vie that the local distiller had made from our crates of pears. This was Father's preferred method for producing Poire Williams, the pear brandy Alsace is famous for, its name taken from the Williams Bon-Chrétien variety (here better known as the Bartlett). Preserved by the alcohol, the pear would last forever, so long as the bottle was refilled every year. My father gave these magical bottles as gifts to relatives or special friends. The bottles always stumped our clever city cousins. At big family reunions the bottle would come out after a four-hour meal so the men could enjoy the obligatory digestif: how had our father got the pear into the bottle? They would squirm a bit, but soon we would reveal how simple it was and how each spring I helped Dad attach the bottle over a budding pear on one of his prime trees. More often than not, the tiny pear would grow as naturally as the others, the bottle permitting plenty of air and sunshine to pass through.

Marvelous as pears are, apples were and are consumed in far greater quantity: in both France and America no fruit is more widely enjoyed. I am a subscriber. I eat at least one apple a day for as long as they are in season, and it's hardly a matter of virtue, since there are so many varieties that I like: Reinette, Golden Delicious, Granny Smith, Mutsu, Boskoop. . . . Their high concentration of antioxidants (especially in the skin) is well known, but I'm convinced that apples help French women avoid getting fat as well. This claim was exploited by a dietitian from Washington State, who proposed a three-apple-a-day diet a couple of years ago. As ever, I don't do or recommend diets, and any strict consumption of three things a day could get monotonous, but there is a nugget of wisdom there. Apples have plenty of fiber for relatively few calories: I can't imagine increasing your consumption of them without achieving a slimming effect, provided you didn't simply add apples to an already overloaded intake. The key to reaping this apple benefit is—big surprise—the pleasure principle: the apple must be full of taste and of an agreeable texture. If the apple has been freshly picked and shipped locally, there's a far better chance that it was picked ripe (not green, for the long haul) and that it won't have lost moisture, the key to crispness. Pears can lose a little water and get sugary; apples only get mealy. If you have an unripe apple, put it in a brown paper bag to be ripened by its naturally emitted ethylene (this also works well for bananas and pears). If you have a ripe one, the best thing to do is eat it. If you must hold it, however, seal it in a food container and refrigerate it. Heresy, I know, putting a fruit in the fridge, but the cold does arrest the ripening process, and the container keeps the apple from drying out. (The same goes for a ripe avocado.) So, while it's always best not to refrigerate fruit, the apple is a rare exception whose life can be extended slightly in the fridge. And if you do refrigerate one, remember to take it out early enough that it can get to room temperature, at which point its flavors will be at their peak, before you eat it. A good apple can be a most satisfying dessert, eaten sliced, with the skin on for the full array of nutrients, and with a knife and fork to make the experience fuller, though still simple and pure. Have you noticed that people tend to chomp on apples without even looking at them? No wonder we were kicked out of the Garden of Eden.

PEAR-APPLE COMPOTE WITH HONEY

Serves 4

INGREDIENTS

1 pound apples
$\frac{2}{3}$ pound pears
Juice of 1 lemon
2 tablespoons honey

1. Peel, core, and dice the apples and pears. Pour lemon juice over them and toss. Into a heavy pan pour $\frac{1}{2}$ cup water and the fruit mixture. Cover and cook over medium heat for 10 minutes, stirring occasionally to prevent the fruit from sticking or burning.

2. With a fork, crush the fruit coarsely while continuing to cook for another 3 to 5 minutes, or until the excess water evaporates. Remove from the heat, add the honey, and mix gently. Serve lukewarm or cold (if you store it in the fridge, take it out 30 minutes before serving).

N.B. PLAY WITH DIFFERENT VARIETIES OF APPLES, PEARS, AND HONEY TO RENEW THE TASTE OF THE COMPOTE. FOR A SPECIAL TREAT, ADD A SMALL SCOOP OF ICE CREAM.

. . . .

JARLSBERG, APPLE, AND MUSHROOM SALAD

Serves 6

1. Sprinkle the mushroom and apple slices with the lemon juice.

2. For dressing: Mix all the dressing ingredients together, seasoning with salt and pepper to taste. Add the mushroom-apple mixture and cheese to the dressing. Toss gently with the lettuce. Serve immediately.

INGREDIENTS

1 pound mushrooms (Crimini go well with the cheese), cleaned and thinly sliced

1 medium Golden Delicious apple, cored and cut into thin slices

3 tablespoons lemon juice

FOR THE DRESSING:

2 tablespoons red wine vinegar

2 tablespoons Meaux mustard

8 tablespoons walnut oil

2 tablespoons freshly chopped parsley

Pinch of curry

Salt and freshly ground pepper

4 ounces Jarlsberg cheese, cut into strips 1 inch long and $\frac{1}{8}$ inch thick

1 large head lettuce, rinsed and dried, leaves torn

N.B. YOU CAN REPLACE LETTUCE WITH MESCLUN OR A VARIETY OF SALAD GREENS, INCLUDING FRISÉE AND ENDIVES.

SPICED APPLES

Serves 4

A nice autumnal accompaniment to white meat, and you can substitute pears if you like. With a little dollop of whipped cream or yogurt, these apples make a nice dessert, too.

INGREDIENTS

2 apples

1 orange

2 tablespoons honey (clover or acacia)

Freshly ground pepper

1. Peel and core the apples and cut each into 8 slices. Cut the unpeeled orange into thin slices. Layer the orange slices in the bottom of a steamer, cover with a layer of apple slices, and end with a layer of orange slices.

2. Steam for 6 to 7 minutes, until the apples are tender and infused with orange perfume. Discard the oranges and serve the apples warm, drizzled with honey. Season with pepper to taste.

· ·

BAKED APPLE AIXOISE

Serves 4

Another Provençal "variation" from my cousin Andrée, the creator of the Provençal version of Magical "Mimosa" Leek Soup. She also loved the family's classic Alsatian recipe for baked apple in French Women Don't Get Fat.

INGREDIENTS

4 Golden Delicious apples

1 Meyer lemon

1. Preheat the oven to 350 degrees.

2. Carefully remove part of each apple's core to form a cavity in the center of the

apple (but not a tunnel through it). Peel the Meyer lemon into strips and reserve the skin.

3. Into each apple put a strip of Meyer lemon skin, a sprig of rosemary, ½ tablespoon of the oil, 1 clove, and ½ tablespoon of the honey.

4. Put the apples in a baking dish and add ⅔ cup water. Cook in the preheated oven for 45 minutes or until the apples start splitting. Serve warm.

INGREDIENTS

4 rosemary sprigs

2 tablespoons olive oil

4 cloves

2 tablespoons lavender honey

. . . .

PEARS WITH CHOCOLATE AND PEPPER

Serves 4

The pear is one of nature's most remarkable inventions; its versatility is second to none. What other fruit could wed so perfectly with chocolate one minute, blue cheese the next?

1. Bring 1 quart water, the orange zest, and the sugar to a boil. Peel and core the pears, keeping them whole by cutting the core out from the bottom, and put them in the boiling syrup over low heat for 20 minutes. Place each pear on a dessert dish and let cool.

INGREDIENTS

Zest of 1 orange

⅔ cup sugar

4 Bosc pears

INGREDIENTS

^{2}/3 cup heavy cream

4 ounces dark chocolate,
coarsely chopped

1 tablespoon unsalted
butter, cut in small pieces

Freshly ground pepper

2. Bring the cream to a boil, then pour in the chocolate and stir to melt it. Whisk in the butter piece by piece. Pour the sauce over the pears and season with pepper to taste. Serve immediately.

N.B. PEPPER IS SURPRISING WITH DESSERT. IT ENHANCES THE FLAVOR OF FRESH FRUIT. IN MY FIRST BOOK, I INCLUDED A PINEAPPLE DESSERT. YOU CAN ALSO USE PEPPER WITH STRAWBERRIES.

. . . .

PEARS ON BRIOCHE

Serves 4

INGREDIENTS

2 ripe pears

1 tablespoon unsalted
butter

4 slices brioche

2 tablespoons honey

2 tablespoons sliced
almonds

1 dollop sour cream or
crème fraîche

1. Preheat the broiler.

2. Peel the pears and cut them into small cubes. Melt the butter in a saucepan and sauté the pear cubes for 2 to 3 minutes over medium-high heat.

3. In a baking dish, arrange the pear cubes on the brioche slices. Cover with the honey and almonds. Put the pan under the preheated broiler for 2 minutes, watching carefully. Serve warm with a dollop of sour cream or crème fraîche.

. . . .

PEAR AND GOAT CHEESE *PAPILLOTE* WITH YOGURT SAUCE

Serves 4

1. Preheat the oven to 350 degrees.

2. Peel the pears, cut them into quarters, and slice each quarter into thirds. Add the lemon juice.

3. Cut 8 pieces of parchment paper (or aluminum foil) into squares large enough to hold 1 ounce of goat cheese and 1 pear's worth of slices and leave a 2-inch border all around. Lightly brush 4 squares of the paper with olive oil. Arrange the pear slices in the center of a square and spread 1 ounce of the goat cheese over each pear. Crumble the blue cheese over the goat cheese and pear slices, drizzle with oil, sprinkle with chervil, and season with salt and pepper to taste.

4. Place the remaining parchment squares on top of the others and fold up the edges to form packets. Simply double folding each of the four sides is enough to seal each packet. Put the *papillotes* on a baking sheet, and bake in the preheated oven for 12 to 15 minutes.

5. For the sauce: Peel the pear, cut it into small pieces, and mix with the yogurt and lemon juice. Season with salt and pepper to taste. Set aside.

INGREDIENTS

4 pears

Juice of 1 lemon

4 ounces fresh goat cheese

2 ounces blue cheese

2 tablespoons olive oil

1 tablespoon fresh chervil or tarragon

Salt and freshly ground pepper

FOR THE SAUCE:

1 pear

1 cup yogurt

Juice of 1 lemon

Salt and freshly ground pepper

6. To serve the *papillotes*, open each packet and slide the contents onto a dish while they are still warm. Serve with your choice of greens and the yogurt sauce on the side.

. . . .

PEARS WITH GINGER AND CHOCOLATE MOUSSE
Serves 4

INGREDIENTS

4 Bosc pears

2 lemons

⅓ cup plus 2 tablespoons sugar, separated

1 teaspoon fresh grated ginger

5 ounces heavy cream

⅓ cup rum

10 ounces dark chocolate, coarsely chopped

1 egg yolk

4 egg whites

1. Peel the pears, keeping them whole, and remove the stems. Put the pears in a saucepan and cover with 2 cups water. Add the zest of 1 lemon, juice of 2 lemons, ⅓ cup of the sugar, and the ginger. Cover and cook over low heat for 15 minutes. Remove the pears and cook the liquid down over medium-high heat until it is reduced to ½ cup of syrup (about 10 minutes). Let cool.

2. For the chocolate mousse, bring the heavy cream to a boil. Stir in the rum and cook for a few minutes. Remove from the heat. Add the chocolate pieces and egg yolk to the cream-rum mixture and combine.

3. Beat the egg whites until firm, adding the 2 tablespoons sugar bit by bit. Mix ⅓ of the egg whites into the chocolate mixture (which should be lukewarm). Fold in the remaining egg whites.

4. Refrigerate the mousse for 2 hours. Serve it as an accompaniment to the gingered pears, drizzled with the reserved syrup.

. . . .

AU CHOCOLAT

If there is any food I look to as compensation for the shortening of days, it is chocolate. Let me be clear: I don't start scarfing it down after Labor Day. But somehow chocolate seems less necessary in summer, besides tending to melt. In fall, and even more so in winter, I depend on it. It must be recognized as potent stuff: potent in taste, potent in nutrients, potent in calories as well. But you don't have to abuse it to enjoy it. A little square savored goes a long way.

My friend Ségolène recently told me that 17 million French people eat chocolate every day, and she is one of them. She takes it always in mid-afternoon, when she feels the need for a little pick-me-up, the operative principle being "little." Chocolate isn't strictly seasonal, so there isn't anything wrong with year-round moderate enjoyment. But as with any pleasure, the experience is heightened by sometimes doing without it. And a basic French woman's rule of weight management is to ask herself how much does she want what she is about to eat. It isn't until fall, when the heat is off meteorologically and the heat is on professionally, that I find my thoughts turning irresistibly toward the dark brown richness of chocolate.

Chocolate is *"ma drogue"* with no negative side effect, and it always puts me in a delicious mood. Considering its effect on the neurotransmitter dopamine as well as its abundance of heart-smart flavonoids (a potent kind of antioxidant), I would advocate that chocolate be covered by health insurance, but that is admittedly a very French public policy perspective. Until that day, when presumably chocolate quality would be regulated as well, it is a good idea to bear in mind that the healthful part is the cocoa content, not the milk fats. For good health, eat the darkest chocolate you can find. Taken sparingly and as needed, you should never get fat from chocolate.

Admittedly, most of us could use some guidance in dosing, as chocolate intake sometimes seems governed by an old fallacy: if a little is good, more must be better. At a book signing on the West Coast, I had just finished reading a passage from the Bread and Chocolate chapter of *French Women Don't Get Fat* when a gentleman approached the lectern to offer me a huge shopping bag I could barely lift filled with an amazing variety of top-quality chocolates. It was obviously a supply for a month even for a serious chocoholic, and little did he know that I was flying to Australia the next day. Yes, I had a fleeting vision of locking myself in my hotel room for a chocolate orgy that night—we all have wicked thoughts, now and again—but fortunately, I was able to gather my wits. I thanked him and told the audience of his beneficence, adding that I knew he wouldn't mind if I shared the gift with everyone at the signing. The applause was thunderous. I'll never forget the sight of this heavenly bounty laid out on the table next to the books, as the line of the devoted (undoubtedly more to chocolate than to me) filed past. Some pieces were bigger than others, the centers held different ganaches, and it was fascinating to observe each person pick out his or her morsel of choice. What except chocolate could bring out both our individuality and the pleasure of sharing?

I always knew the best chocolate moments are not *"en cachette"* (on the sly), but as a communal treat, with friends or family, especially at the end of a meal. Special occasions like a birthday or anniversary, or other joyous times, can be honored with chocolate, though as I discovered, anywhere two or more people relish chocolate together can be a special occasion.

Even in fall and winter many chocolate confections are better enjoyed on their own, but I sometimes do indulge in them for dessert, provided the meal has not been on the heavy side. I like chocolate desserts that combine hot and cold, such as *profiteroles au chocolat:* the dark warm chocolate sauce and the cold vanilla ice cream colliding in luscious sweetness cut by the dough of the *pâte à choux.* More often I enjoy the way deep, dark chocolate marries with fruits—strawberries, raspberries, and cherries, but also pears and oranges, prunes, dried apricots, and dates—or with nuts, including pecans, pistachios, and my supreme favorite, chestnuts. My mother's *Ardèchois au chocolat et marrons* is a living memory in taste, image, and spirit.

When I invite people for dinner at home, I usually make two desserts, and one has to be chocolate. At the beginning of my married life, we often had dinner for six in our Greenwich Village apartment. One time we had invited some of Edward's college friends whom I barely knew, and, as usual, the last course included chocolate, in this case a flourless chocolate cake with a bit of whipped cream. I served a small piece to each of our guests and offered no seconds at the end of a rather long and elaborate dinner. As the last couple was leaving later in the evening, I noticed Edward's buddy John eyeing (actually, more nearly devouring with his eyes) the remaining half of the chocolate cake, which was resting on the kitchen counter. We were leaving for Europe the following night, so I offered to let him and his wife take it home for the weekend. The next morning, John phoned to thank us for dinner and especially for the incredible chocolate cake, which he had eaten on the way home (an hour's drive outside the city)—he couldn't remember eating anything so good. What could I say? I felt a bit of guilt, having led him into temptation. Next time I would remember that friends don't let friends who aren't French women drive with half a chocolate cake.

FLOURLESS CHOCOLATE CAKE

Serves 8

I always prefer this cake the next day. It's a perfect, rich dessert for cool weather. There is no need to refrigerate it—just cover loosely with waxed paper and keep it in a cool place. If refrigerated, make sure to take it out at least 2 hours before serving.

INGREDIENTS

8 ounces dark chocolate

8 ounces unsalted butter, at room temperature, plus extra for buttering pan

4 large eggs

1 cup sugar

¼ cup Grand Marnier or orange-flavored liqueur

6 tablespoons cornstarch

1. Preheat the oven to 350 degrees. Brush a 4-cup ring mold or a 9-inch springform pan with butter.

2. Chop the chocolate and melt it in a bowl set above a simmering pan of water. Remove and let cool. While the chocolate is cooling, cream the butter in a mixing bowl.

3. Pour the cooled, melted chocolate into the mixing bowl with the butter and beat for 2 minutes. The mixture should be thick. Set aside.

4. In a separate bowl, beat the eggs. Start adding the sugar, beating at high speed, until the eggs are thick and very pale yellow (6 to 8 minutes). Both the egg-sugar and chocolate-butter mixtures should have a similar consistency.

5. Beat the chocolate-butter mixture into the egg-sugar mixture and add the Grand Marnier. Beat another minute to mix. Sift the cornstarch into the batter and gently fold in.

6. Pour the batter into the prepared mold. Tap the mold on the counter to level and cover with buttered waxed paper. Put the mold in a baking dish and fill the dish with near-boiling water, almost up to the top of the mold. Put the baking dish with the mold in the preheated oven for 45 to 50 minutes. Let cool. Turn upside down on a serving platter, but wait 30 minutes to remove the mold.

7. Serve with unsugared whipped cream.

. . . .

We are all adults, and therefore we are ultimately responsible for our respective indulgences. We have to learn restraint so we know how to face a shopping bag full of great chocolate or half a flourless chocolate cake. As ever, the key to eating a proper amount is really enjoying what you do eat: gluttony is a desperate bid to satisfy our head, not our stomach. You know you are really eating for pleasure when you surprise yourself by having less than you expected.

And sometimes by just saying no. A few years ago, I was

invited to a holiday-theme lunch at a famous food magazine with the top brass. When coffee was served (and it's only after a special lunch that I would have coffee during the day after breakfast), out came the chocolate truffles. They looked divine, and I decided to savor one with my coffee. Conversation was animated, and before I knew it the platter was circulating a second time with some people already eating their third truffle. But one small bite of the first one was enough to tell me these truffles were not very good, let alone first-rate. I discreetly left the rest on my saucer. An observer might have imagined I was exercising astonishing self-control, but it was really quite easy to pass on something that offered little or no pleasure. With the holidays approaching, I knew I would be eating truly irresistible chocolate before long. I didn't mind waiting.

We do get a little careless at this time of year, because so many "goodies" are put before us, even if many of them are not so good. It also seems that the remoteness of bikini season gives many of us license to let ourselves go and take cover under less revealing clothes. But that only sets you up to face losing weight in springtime. Sure, it happens, but there is no need to regard fall/winter weight gain as inevitable. If you tend your equilibrium, eating for pleasure and mindful of taste and choice, you can enjoy the season without fear of getting fat. Anyway, clothes should not be a way of concealing ourselves but of flattering ourselves.

As many women will admit, there is no better time of year for wearing clothes. Not that they would otherwise be topless: it's merely that in fall we can wear things without feeling as if we're overbundled or a sweaty mess. Springtime, too, is this way in theory, but in many places one goes straight into summer dress. The spring coat, so common until the sixties and still favored by the ultra chic, has alas become an anachronism for most. People today seem to revel in going out wearing as little as they can. When I see kids at New England schools and universities wearing shorts at the first sign of the winter thaw, I imagine a sort of pagan invocation of warmth. I mind that much less than those unseasonably skimpy styles that just won't go away. Let's draw a veil over those, or at least a scarf.

Even for those not scantily clad, scarves really are indispensable for fall. Paired with a simple quilted jacket of nylon or microfiber, they always create a faultlessly chic and affordable outdoor look. (And a French woman would make sure the jacket line, or any other, doesn't end at some point on her body to which she would rather not draw attention.) I am not much of an American varsity football fan, but I've always adored the look of those college and school scarves, which, over a jacket, provide just enough warmth in autumn. Personally, in the fall, I like to wear scarves like long necklaces, which can be transformed into stoles to take a dress into evening. As in summer, a uniform of simple trim-fitting sheath dresses and a few neutral skirts and sweaters of good quality can provide a base. There's always a jacket or some other single piece you can buy to get the current look, while keeping all else mostly timeless.

Long Necklace Scarf

You'll need a rectangular scarf long enough so that each end reaches down to your belt when it hangs around your neck.

1. Fold the scarf in half once or twice depending on its width.
2. With the scarf around your neck, take one length and loop it into a simple knot that hangs just above your first rib.

3. Pull the other end through the loop and then tighten the loop knot, adjusting the two lengths so they are even and the knot is well positioned.

Side-knotted Oblong Scarf

This knot and style have become very fashionable. A short scarf works best over a sweater and a longer version over a jacket or coat.

1. Fold an oblong scarf in half lengthwise and then double by bringing both of the long ends together (like a rope).
2. Place it around your neck and pull the folded loop end across to one side of your body and pass the other end of the scarf through the loop.
3. Pull down on the hanging end to tighten for comfort and positioning off-center.

Shoulder Wrap

This is a quick trick for so-called French elegance par excellence. It requires a glorious scarf that goes with a solid-colored dress.

1. Fold diagonally in half to create a triangle.
2. Place the scarf over one shoulder and pull the two long ends across your body (one behind and one in front) and knot the ends just above the hip opposite the shoulder upon which the scarf rests.

It's very easy and typical in fall to take our color cues from the landscape. Heathery and brownish tweeds, deep rust and golden woolens are unimpeachable and these colors usually look too drab or edgy in spring and summer. While these colors are flattering and easy to wear, there is no necessity of banishing bright color in fall. Often one bright saturated color can fetchingly offset the sobriety of other clothes and if you pick the color of the season (fashion's, not the earth's), you needn't make much more effort to look au courant.

• A Week's Menu for Fall •

MONDAY

Breakfast

½ cup Grandma Louise's
    Oatmeal with Grated
    Apple (www
    .mireilleguiliano.com)
⅓ cup milk
½ teaspoon brown sugar
1 slice of sourdough bread,
    toasted and buttered
Coffee or tea

Lunch

Jarlsberg, Apple, and Mush-
    room Salad (page 173)
1 seven-grain roll
1 square chocolate
Noncaloric beverage

Dinner

Skate with Capers
    (page 164)
Cauliflower Gratin
    (page 157)
½ cup greens
½ cup yogurt
1 pear
1 glass white or red wine

TUESDAY

Breakfast

1 teaspoon soy nuts
2-egg omelet
1 slice whole wheat bread,
    toasted and buttered
½ grapefruit
Coffee or tea

Lunch

1 cup Basic Vegetable Soup
    (www.mireilleguiliano
    .com)
1 slice country bread
½ cup yogurt
1 apple
Noncaloric beverage

Dinner

Macaroni with Pancetta
    (page 162)
½ cup broccoli rabe
Mango Carpaccio with
    Cinnamon (page 231)
1 glass red wine

• A Week's Menu for Fall •

WEDNESDAY

Breakfast

½ cup yogurt
1 kiwi
1 small brioche or half a
    bagel with butter and jam
Coffee or tea

Lunch

Chicken and Haricots Verts
    Salad (page 163)
6 almonds
1 cup black grapes
Noncaloric beverage

Dinner

Cod with Potato Salad
    (page 155)
½ cup spinach
Sautéed Mushrooms
    (page 78)
Crème caramel
1 glass white or red wine

THURSDAY

Breakfast

2 prunes
½ cup freshly squeezed
    grapefruit juice or
    ½ grapefruit
½ cup yogurt
1 fried egg
1 slice whole wheat bread,
    toasted and buttered
Coffee or tea

Lunch

1 cup Green Soup (page 112)
1 slice black olive roll or
    whole wheat bread
1 ounce cheese
½ papaya
Noncaloric beverage

Dinner

Pork Chops with Apples
    (www.mireilleguiliano
    .com)
⅓ cup brown rice
Mixed salad
Mousse au Chocolat
    (www.mireilleguiliano
    .com)
1 glass white or red wine

• A Week's Menu for Fall •

Breakfast

1 ounce cheese
1 slice prosciutto
1 soft-boiled egg
1 slice seven-grain bread,
    toasted and buttered
3 dried apricots
Coffee or tea

Lunch

Buttersquash Soup
    (page 159)
1 cup green veggies
½ banana
Noncaloric beverage

Dinner

Turkey Scaloppine with
    Pesto (page 166)
½ cup mashed potatoes
Green salad
Pear-Apple Compote with
    Honey (page 172)
1 glass red wine

Breakfast

1 slice boiled ham
½ cup freshly squeezed
    orange juice or 1 orange
½ cup oatmeal with raisins
    and walnuts
½ cup milk
Coffee or tea

Lunch

Mussels in White Wine
    (page 165)
1 slice country bread
Mâche salad with 1 ounce
    nuts and a pear
Noncaloric beverage

Dinner

Grilled Steak with Wine
    Sauce (page 167)
1 baked potato with butter or
    sour cream
Green salad
1 slice chocolate cake
1 glass red wine

• A Week's Menu for Fall •

Breakfast

½ cup yogurt
Pears on Brioche (page 176)
Coffee or tea

Lunch (main meal)

Seafood platter (oysters,
    crab, and clams)
1 slice rye bread with salted
    butter
1 cup green veggies
Baked Apple Aixoise
    (page 174)
1 glass Champagne or
    sparkling wine

Dinner

1 cup Celeriac Soup
    (page 211)
½ cup carrots, sautéed
½ cup raw fennel
1 ounce hard cheese
½ grapefruit

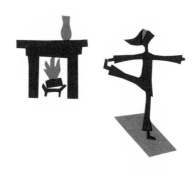

5

Most of us really don't have the choice to sit winter out. The fact is that not every bird gets to fly south. And I confess I wouldn't want to: I love my morning walks in the winter, breathing the cool, crisp air, and I can't imagine living in places without much seasonal variation. When the passing of the year doesn't impress itself upon my senses, I am, in some profound sense, lost.

As the days shorten, other mammals grow fuller coats and change color. Let's not kid ourselves: winter has an effect on us as well. In the northern climes, including Paris and New York, a point comes when it seems the cold and long hours indoors will never end, when the snows of two months ago are often still piled in the streets, and nothing is left in the cupboard but a few shriveled root vegetables. Okay, *j'exagère,* but you know the feeling. There is scant comfort in knowing that it's worse elsewhere: Buffalo gets almost 100 inches of snow a year. Or consider Sweden, an enchanting land in the summer, when the sun rises at 3 a.m., but where in winter there are but four brief hours of gray so-called daylight. No, the real consolation is in knowing what awaits us when it's over: the regeneration of everything in spring. I'm not just looking on the bright side here. I would not trade that thrill, and that awareness of progress—of the fullness of time—for the eternal sunshine of a spotless mind in L.A.

Christmas is celebrated in December less because we believe the Nativity actually occurred then and more as a perpetuation of ancient rites designed to bring some light into the darkness. But once the unwanted gifts have been returned and the last cork of New Year's has been popped, we enter a bit of a tunnel. With relatively little light and even less fresh unfattening food to enjoy—and having perhaps allowed an extra pound or two to creep aboard during the holidays—we are more vulnerable than ever to getting fat. What can we do to keep it all together? In fact, there is plenty. We need not—and after all, we cannot—spend those months when the slant of light oppresses simply huddled under the duvet with a book, much as a French woman delights in doing that sometimes.

In winter many of us rise in darkness and return home from work in darkness, practically never having seen the light of day. There's a reason nature has designed some animals to sleep through the whole affair. We, however, aren't so lucky—or perhaps we are luckier. Winter's purpose is to clear the decks so nature can start over. Long ago, a person's age would be expressed by how many winters she had on her back. Now technology spares us the worst effects of the elements; the rest is up to us. The trick is to make it as full and energetic a period as it can be.

First, let us acknowledge that humans, like bears and birds, are photoperiodic: we are affected by the duration of daylight. Most of us experience to some degree what has come to be called Seasonal Affective Disorder. In other words, the dearth of light brings us down. And many of us take refuge from the blahs in food. *Qu'est-ce qu'on va faire?* One simple solution is to make a point of going outside at midday. If you work in an office, your exposure to light in winter can easily be limited to the fluorescent variety, which is neither flattering nor healthy. Take a little break at noon and soak up what sunshine you can. (A French woman—at least this French woman—will still wear sunglasses to avoid squinting in the glare and crow's-feet.) This exposure can help keep our sleep cycles in order— the disruption of these is one of winter's biggest health risks. It also gives you some chance of producing the vitamin D your body requires, although in winter it must be supplemented by tablet and by D-rich foods such as milk, egg yolks, and tuna.

Even on the gloomiest days, a lunchtime promenade will do you good, for the other compensation for the lack of light is to move. Apart from its metabolic and cardiovascular benefits, physical exertion is known to have a stimulative effect on the neurotransmitters that keep our spirits up. Snow sports have become hugely popular in the last few years. Many people I know track the months of winter by the ski season. But just mention the word *ski* and I imagine not the amazing rush but the prospect of chapped skin in bone-chilling cold, killer trees, and broken bones (mine). Fine for the ski set, not for me, though I do encourage sportier types at least in the less hair-raising cross-country version. Or ice-skating! (In Paris, Rollerblading en masse seems to continue *sans interruption* on weekends through the winter.) Any exercise we undertake for pleasure is a good one. I am told the gym serves as a refuge for some in the winter. But even sans skis and Cybex, I find lots of easy ways of getting my heart rate up and working my muscles, overcoming the ever-present temptation to sleep in.

So what do I do? Walking and yoga are my prime winter movements. After the metabolic slowdown of winter sleep, it's important not just to get the body going but to awaken the mind to the body. Feel the connection—it's my French Zen thing. Some simple stretching before breakfast can do wonders. In New York, I leave the house by taking the stairs down fourteen floors. That wakes my body up for sure. And when I don't get as much movement in my normal day as I'd like, I make a point of taking the stairs back up . . . often all the way to the fifteenth floor. In winter, the stairs really can be the most efficient and convenient way of elevating not just yourself but your heart rate and mood. And you can avoid hypothermia: New York, for example, can be wickedly cold on winter mornings. On the subfreezing days when I see those morning joggers trailing vapor from their mouths and noses, I have to smile. They don't need to do that to be healthy. I hope they are doing it for pleasure. I imagine these people must be skiers, too.

Though sometimes it is just too cold and windy to leave the house, I do love to walk in the snow . . . especially in New York City. New York with its clear blue winter skies and buzzing streets can become transcendentally quiet when a thick white blanket is first laid down. The traffic disappears (save the large sanitation trucks transformed into plows). Edward and I look forward to heading out after a blizzard for a long walk. Like walking on the edge of the surf on the beach, trudging through fresh snow is wonderful exercise and, as every kid knows, great fun. As we walk down the center of big avenues and little side streets, passing fellow travelers, the streetscape feels as it must have centuries ago. Everything is still and clean, and the community becomes a picturesque village of children on sleds (an odd thing to find in Manhattan, but you do) and neighbors shoveling the sidewalks . . . eventually some begin to dig out their cars, only to have them partially reburied by the plows. Everyone seems in high spirits, even—perhaps especially—those shovelers. The stores slowly reopen, and people share in the wintry gift of a small reprieve from the demands of schedule.

Winter rain is something else, though. It can be awful, and I certainly don't walk in it for pleasure or exercise, though the humid air is wonderful for the skin; on dry winter days, both skin and hair need moisturizing. An excellent homemade beauty mask of *Mamie*'s is always at the ready. She was big on these natural treatments, and in the winter, once a week she'd cut a slice of lemon or grapefruit and rub it on her face first thing in the morning. It was her trick to clarify the top layer of the skin. For my teenage pre-period skin problems, she'd put some parsley juice on a piece of cotton and apply it to troublesome spots. For the oily and dull skin of my cousin, she'd mix some grapes with almonds and apply the paste to her face (use your coffee grinder or a blender to do the mixing), leaving it on for a few minutes and rinsing with cold water. Egg mixtures were some of the most effective weapons in her arsenal. No matter the skin type, she'd recommend this one over and over: before a party, mix an egg yolk with a few drops of olive oil and leave the mixture on the face for 15 minutes. Another one was a mixture of an egg yolk, a few lettuce leaves, and ½ cup of yogurt; it tightens the pores and hydrates the skin. Concocting something soothing for your face can make an afternoon at home feel like a day at the spa. (Speaking of spas, massages are cheaper and easier to come by these days, and they can be a great way of pampering yourself.) But in any case, make yourself a pitcher of lemon water, get out your yoga mat, and after some poses treat yourself to a mask. I have been doing yoga year-round for decades, but in winter I double up at home and love to take classes to expand my practice. In yoga, as in life, one is always learning.

The house gives me another outlet of exertion, this one productive as well as healthful. Even French women with French maids like to *faire le ménage.* Other Europeans, too. Recently the *Wall Street Journal* reported that the least effective way to market cleaning products to Italian women is to tout their time-saving convenience. It would seem the Italians know what French women do: convenience has its downside. We are too quick to write off and evade as drudgery activities that keep the blood flowing while giving us a small but satisfying sense of accomplishment. We all need such a sense in this world we've created, where the goals we set ourselves can be so complex.

Finally, I have a little anti-stress winter exercise that makes me feel good physically and mentally, whether I'm at home or at work. Have you ever picked low-hanging fruit from a tree? Apples, cherries, peaches, pears, whatever? Imagine yourself standing under that tree and reaching up as high as you can with one arm to pluck a ripe fruit. Are you on your toes? Got it? Great. Now place it in a basket at your feet. Relax and breathe deeply. Now reach up with your other arm and stretch for another fruit, then bend and place it in the basket. Alternate arms until you have filled the basket with twenty or more pieces of fruit. Got more time, need more exercise or escape? Move to a different fruit tree and repeat. Apart from triggering the release of neurotransmitters that create a sense of *bien-être* (well-being), exercises like this loosen tight muscles and bring oxygen-rich blood to the brain, helping to reduce high levels of cortisol, the hormone associated with stress (and not surprisingly with the storage of body fat). For me, just thinking about being outdoors under a fruit tree is a soothing mental vacation in time and space. It's a lot cheaper than Palm Beach, and I can just taste those fruits.

PRÊT-À-CHAUFFER

Imagining yourself in the orange grove, you might prefer to be wearing a sundress, but otherwise we must take account of the elements when we put ourselves together in winter. If we let the downside of the season overwhelm us, we can easily get frumpy, hiding under our outer garments and bulky sweaters. A French woman must look soignée, pulled together. Her clothes must flatter her shape without obscuring it or baring too much. What goes the rest of the year for cut and quality goes in winter as well: buy to fit, not to billow or constrict, and buy simple basics of quality before all else. Buy chic navies, blacks, beiges, and grays and play colors off against them.

The winter's "interview suit," which is the everyday suit in law firms and in the federal government, is fortunately receding as the business standard. A nicely tailored jacket can go a long way, creating a polished, professional look with a blouse and trousers. Fragrance is also indispensable to me in winter, when I like something spicy or woodsy. There are many nice florals, too, and with the weather colder, I don't mind wearing something a little more complex.

Not surprisingly, I consider winter scarves as much an element of style as of warmth. Obviously, any scarf style can be worn during any season, but in winter I like to keep my neck wrapped, whether wearing the scarf over a dress, blouse, or coat. Silk can be remarkably warm, but lambswool and cashmere are the winter fibers of choice. Nowadays a warm cashmere shawl (ideal for a wrap over a coat) has become an affordable luxury item, widely available and no longer forbiddingly expensive.

Neck-Wrap Scarf

If you have a long neck, this choker style is especially elegant (and warm) under a coat and over a sweater, blouse, or dress.

1. Take a rectangular scarf and fold it in half lengthwise once or twice.
2. Put it around your neck with the ends toward your back, wrap it around the front of your neck and around to the back again.
3. Tie it, tucking loose ends under the wrap.

Ascot-Bib Scarf

1. Fold a square scarf in half diagonally to create a triangle.
2. With the point of the triangle hanging under your chin, pull the two ends over your shoulders, crossing the ends at the back of your neck then drawing them to the front under your chin. Tie in front with a simple knot.

Knotless Over-the-Shoulder Wrap

If there's no wind, this wrap works well over a coat to create an extra layer of insulation and especially to cover your throat.

1. Fold a large square or rectangular scarf in half horizontally.
2. Place it around your neck and pull down one end to make it at least six inches longer than the other side. Toss the long end up and over your opposite shoulder, making sure the body of the scarf drapes and covers your upper chest and neck. Adjust as appropriate. You can also pin this scarf in front with a brooch or light, ornamental stickpin.

BONNE DÉGUSTATION

Okay, so your blood is flowing and you are dressed for success. But what's to eat? Even more than in autumn, I need chocolate. If in autumn I feel there should be a prescription drug benefit covering chocolate, in winter I find myself advocating a national strategic chocolate reserve, so convinced am I of its consoling powers. But we still have to observe moderation. Even in winter, or rather in winter especially, we must fashion a plan of nourishment suited to the demands on our bodies, as well as to the limited variety of foodstuffs. Life can't all be treats, but it should still be filled with pleasures, so let me begin with the ones most deeply ingrained in my own psyche.

The first word in winter food worldwide tends to be the dishes served at feasts that have carried over from the earliest pagan celebrations of the solstice. The food is typically elaborate, and these convivial occasions are often the last chance to gather loved ones together until the thaw. The fear that first inspired these rites—fear that the failing light would never return unless we propitiated the gods—has itself mostly faded, but the French have never needed an excuse to pop a cork or share a meal. There are four gastronomic pillars of the typical French holiday menu, especially for Christmas: chestnuts, oysters, turkey, and the ubiquitous *bûche de Noël* or Yule log.

MARRONS

In our kitchen on frosty weekend evenings starting mid-December, my mother would bring out a small wicker basket covered with a cloth napkin under which was a mound of raw chestnuts. We knew we were in for a treat. She would score them with a small sharp knife and set them in a skillet on top of the stove to roast as we eagerly waited. That scent in the kitchen was always linked to Christmas and the holiday season, particularly as *Mamie* would often also bake on those evenings. When the chestnuts were ready, the challenge was to peel them while they were still warm without burning our fingers. That danger was part of the fun, and the first kid to cry "*aïe!*" might need the adults to come to the rescue. It often happened to me since I was unable to peel them as fast as I could eat them, the membranes clinging to the flesh, especially in the crevices of the multifruited kind.

Later, as a student in Paris, I discovered the big-city version of my childhood Yuletide madeleine: street-corner charcoal braziers in Saint-Germain or the Champs-Élysées or any main intersection, often near movie theaters for those leaving the show. We would buy chestnuts freshly roasted, still warm in bags fashioned of layered newspaper. They were neither as good nor as hot as those I remembered from home. But they were a treat all the same, and an affordable one. To this day, whether outside the department stores in Paris, such as the BHV, or on Madison Avenue in midtown Manhattan, it is hard for me to pass up a few warm chestnuts—one of the few truly wholesome street foods.

Of course, there were more elaborate and fancy ways of eating chestnuts as part of holiday meals. Sometimes they would be proffered in a rich soup, my favorites being a velvety cream of celery finished off with pieces of bacon and roasted chestnuts or the luscious and luxurious little tasting cup of chestnut cream soup. Sometimes the big chestnuts would simply be slow-roasted as a vegetable accompaniment to game dishes, particularly *pintade* (guinea hen), pheasant, and venison.

But my most cherished discovery of this seasonal delight took place in Provence, where chestnuts are part of the "after dessert." Nowadays big events have "after parties"; but for as long as I can remember, big meals in France have always had the "after desserts" called petits fours—bite-sized pastries and chocolates. These would be served with the coffee, which follows dessert. *Marrons glacés*, or glazed chestnuts, are not actually frozen, but they are supremely sweet and delicious, my choice for the queen of after desserts when you are pulling out all the stops. They have become the object of some very opinionated connoisseurship in Paris.

My Uncle Charles gave me a lesson in the art of *marrons glacés*, which he had mastered. Like everything in cooking, the quality begins with the ingredients: impeccable chestnuts come from Torino in Italy (the very best are enormous and of silken texture), or Naples or Collobrières in the French Var, and even the Ardèche, where my uncle had his restaurant in a spa town. The big and perfect specimens that passed muster were boiled till tender and would be ever so lightly dipped in crystallized ice-sugar syrup so as to produce just a patina of glazing while the chestnut within remained *moelleux* (soft). Each would then be wrapped in gold foil. I will confess that very few people make their own, though the quest for perfection can be a long one. I can report my own has ended happily at Stohrer, the high temple of gourmandise in the second arrondissement in Paris; many other chestnut freaks concur. When you bite into one perhaps you'll see stars, as Dom Pérignon claimed when first tasting Champagne—at least I do. A purveyor of similar sublimity is Pierre Marcolini, a world-class *chocolatier*, located down the street from our Paris apartment and now also in New York City (talk about temptation!). Nothing says "I love you" at Christmas like his little four-pack of *marrons glacés*. It's also the gift of confidence in one's appreciation of moderation. They will keep at peak flavor for just a few weeks, but one should never eat more than one at a time. Okay, never say never.

CHESTNUTS AND HONEY

Serves 4

INGREDIENTS

1 pound chestnuts

2 tablespoons acacia honey

Salt and freshly ground pepper

1. Peel the chestnuts and cook in boiling water until tender, about 20 minutes. Drain and pat dry.

2. Warm the honey in a large pan over medium heat and add the chestnuts, stirring to coat. Stir until they have caramelized slightly. Season with salt and pepper to taste.

N.B. SERVE THIS WITH ANY WINTER BIRD SUCH AS TURKEY, PHEASANT, OR GUINEA HEN.

. . . .

CHESTNUT SOUP

Serves 4

INGREDIENTS

1 pound peeled chestnuts (jars of peeled chestnuts can be purchased at most finer grocery stores)

2 to 3 cups beef or vegetable stock

½ cup heavy cream

Salt and freshly ground pepper

1 tablespoon unsalted butter

2 tablespoons minced parsley

1. Put the peeled chestnuts in a saucepan with 2 cups of the stock. Bring to a simmer, uncovered, for 40 to 50 minutes, adding more stock, if necessary, to keep the chestnuts covered.

2. When the chestnuts are tender, drain, reserving the stock. Purée the chestnuts in a food processor or blender. Return the puréed chestnuts to the reserved stock, stirring, and add in the heavy cream. Season with salt and pepper to taste. Just before serving add the butter and parsley.

. . . .

Did I tell you I love oysters? I mean, I really love oysters and eat them often. And they are good for you—low in calories and high in nutritional value. When I was growing up, we followed the prescription of eating oysters only in months with *r*'s in them, as that was both when they were harvested and when it was cool enough to ship them safely. Today, with oyster farms and modern transportation, refrigeration, and global shipping, it is possible to eat them year-round. Cold, juicy oysters can be a summer treat, but as a true French woman, they speak winter to me (and fall and spring). Farmed oysters are not significantly inferior to the wild kind—a very different case from, say, salmon. In fact, oyster aquaculture is sustainable and eco-friendly, and so with a fastidious supplier you may do better than with some who troll oyster beds at sea— certainly in the warmer months, when I don't advise eating them raw. Still, oysters are such a staple in late fall and winter, and such a winter holiday tradition in France—just writing this, I can taste Brittany's fine Claire and Belon varieties on the half shell and see the men on New Year's Eve shucking them by the dozen at temporary stands on Paris market streets—I don't feel the need to eat them except in the natural course of their lives, so long as that ends in my stomach. Starting in December, the French eat them raw or cooked, though the latter is, of course, the only sensible way to use them in a stuffing.

Over the past decade as raw seafood bars have become common in restaurants, Americans have come to appreciate oysters more. That's smart: despite such a luscious taste and texture, oysters are not fattening, up to the first couple of dozen anyway. A bit like wine, oysters come in different types and styles typical of their *terroir*, insofar as one can speak of a *terroir*—localized soil and climate—in water. Drawing in countless gallons of local water and nutrients as its sweet flesh plumpens, the oyster is very much a product of where it spawns, and two of the same variety raised in two different locations won't taste the same. In America, there are wonderful kinds from both the East Coast (from Maine to Delaware) and the West. My favorite is the tiny Kumamoto oyster from the Pacific Northwest, which I enjoy whenever I can at Balthazar, a restaurant in New York's SoHo. Perhaps I should have been born a century ago when New York City was the oyster capital of the world and Restaurant Prunier in Paris had an entire menu with oysters!

In America we still don't have the selection found in France, which is Europe's largest producer, with 200 kinds and a yield of 120,000 tons a year, mostly for domestic consumption. (The connection with French men as great lovers has never been proved, but the concentration of zinc, vital for prostate health, does make me wonder.) Such variety presents delicious possibilities when going to a restaurant with friends; with each person ordering a different kind, everyone can have a *dégustation d'huîtres*—an oyster tasting menu. You can compare flavors between the two basic kinds: on the one hand the *plates* (flat), such as Belons (powerful and *iodées*—tasting of the sea) and Marennes (a more refined taste); on the other hand, the *creuses* (convex), such as Portuguaises, Boudeuses (pouters), and including *les fines* (small and delicate) and *les spéciales* (fleshy).

To test your connoisseurship further, some restaurants

offer "boutique oysters" with the name of the grower listed on the menu. My weakness is for Giraudeau, and I'm lucky to be near the wonderful restaurant-brasserie Alcazar in the sixth arrondissement, which becomes my cafeteria during winter stays in Paris and which always seems to carry Giraudeau's offerings on the menu. Regardless of variety, however, oysters are rich in protein, minerals, and vitamins. If you haven't made a place for them in your life, they are a most consoling discovery in winter.

"As I ate the oysters, with their strong taste of the sea and their faint metallic taste that the cold white wine washed away, leaving only the sea taste and the succulent texture, as I drank their cold liquid from each shell and washed it down with the crisp taste of the wine, I lost the empty feeling and began to be happy and to make plans." That's how Ernest Hemingway had them in his memoir of Paris in the 1920s, *A Moveable Feast*. That's how they have been enjoyed for centuries. As far as I am concerned, when serving oysters on the half shell, you can hold the mignonette (that's the classic dressing of shallots and vinegar served in French bistros), and if you are serving them warm, the same goes even for the caviar that sometimes dots them. All you need is a few drops of lemon juice (especially if some of the exquisite liquid has been lost), and if your taste runs like mine, a touch of freshly ground pepper. Add some thin slices of rye bread with salted butter and it's a feast. WWHD (What Would Hemingway Drink)? Champagne is festive and always appropriate, Sauvignon Blanc is totally correct, but more often than not I opt for the inexpensive but so perfectly matched Muscadet from the Loire Valley.

If your palate is new to oysters, a warm preparation is an easy introduction. They are divine with leeks (as recommended in the leek section); spinach is a close second, but all are easy, so feel free to experiment. If opening them intimidates you more than eating them, your fishmonger will be glad to do it. He will put the oyster and its liquid in a container and gladly give you the empty shells if the recipe presentation requires them.

COCKTAIL D'HUÎTRES

Serves 4

INGREDIENTS

12 oysters
½ cup apple juice
Juice of 1 lemon
1 Granny Smith apple, peeled, cored, and cubed

1. Open and drain the oysters, reserving their liquid for another use, perhaps a soup (if your fishmonger opens the oysters for you, ask him to give you the liquid, too). Put 3 oysters in each of 4 martini glasses.

2. Put the apple juice, lemon juice, and a few cubes of the apple in a bowl. Mix well and distribute over the oysters. Serve immediately.

N.B. AN OYSTER KNIFE MAKES IT EASY TO OPEN OYSTERS, AND A THICK RUBBER GLOVE MAKES IT SAFE. OYSTERS CAN BE PURCHASED ALREADY SHUCKED.

. . . .

OYSTER SOUP

Serves 4

Today's cutting-edge chefs are getting very creative with amazing combinations. As always, some work better than others. But the soupe au lait d'huîtres *at* Maison de Bricourt *in Normandy was an experience worth the detour. And it has inspired this version of mine.*

1. Open the oysters, remove from shells, and poach them in a mixture of oyster water (liquor) and butter over low heat for 3 to 5 minutes, until they swell and their thin edges start curling.

2. Add the milk and paprika and season with salt and pepper to taste. Bring to a boil, then cook over low heat, stirring occasionally, for 10 to 12 minutes. Serve immediately with buttered toast.

INGREDIENTS

24 oysters, with their liquor

2 tablespoons unsalted butter

1 quart milk (regular or 2 percent)

1 teaspoon paprika

Salt and freshly ground pepper

. . . .

OYSTERS WITH GARLIC BUTTER

Serves 4

1. Preheat the broiler.

2. Put the butter in a bowl. Press the garlic cloves over the butter and mix well. Add the parsley, season with salt and pepper to taste, and refrigerate.

INGREDIENTS

6 tablespoons unsalted butter, at room temperature

2 cloves garlic, peeled

4 tablespoons minced parsley

Salt and freshly ground pepper

INGREDIENTS

24 oysters
Coarse salt for baking sheet

3. Open the oysters and put them, in their shells, on a baking sheet filled with coarse salt. Add about ½ teaspoon of the parsley-butter mixture to each oyster and broil for 1 to 2 minutes. Serve immediately with rye bread.

. . . .

OYSTERS WITH LEMON ZEST

Serves 4

INGREDIENTS

24 oysters, with their liquor
2 shallots, peeled but whole
6 tablespoons unsalted butter, cut into pieces
Coarse salt for baking sheet
Zest of 1 lemon
Freshly ground pepper

1. Preheat the broiler.

2. Open the oysters, remove them from the shells, and set aside, reserving their liquor.

3. Strain the liquor (you should have ¾ to 1 cup) to remove any stray pieces of shell. Bring the liquid and shallots to a boil. Continue cooking until reduced by half. Remove the shallots and whisk in the butter. Keep the sauce warm on top of a pan of simmering water or in a double boiler.

4. Put the oysters back in their shells and place them on a baking sheet filled with coarse salt, which will keep them in place. Sprinkle the oysters with lemon zest, some

of the sauce, and season with pepper to taste. Broil until golden, 1 to 2 minutes. Serve immediately with a baguette to soak up the delicious juice.

. . . .

SOUPS

Let's face it, in winter we find ourselves scraping for fresh vegetables. Passing these months without an arsenal of canned Italian tomato paste is inconceivable. But as in all seasons, soup is an unsurpassed way of eating a good serving of what is fresh as well as what keeps. Early in winter, for instance, celeriac, a deliciously nutty bulb related to celery, is available for a short time, and I never fail to take advantage. It really is good only in season.

CELERIAC SOUP

Serves 6

As in their mashed potatoes recipe, the women in my family love to experiment with the ratio of potato to celeriac in soup, always in favor of the latter it seems, and, of course, they can't help adding some leeks. When in Provence, we add a drizzle of olive oil for that extra—I'll say it only this once—"je ne sais quoi." It makes me love this soup even more.

INGREDIENTS

2 tablespoons olive oil

1 pound celeriac, peeled
and cubed

¾ pound potatoes, peeled
and cubed

1 leek, white part only,
sliced

2 onions, peeled and
minced

2 shallots, minced

4 cups vegetable stock

1 bay leaf

Salt and freshly ground
pepper

1 cup milk (regular or
2 percent)

6 slices of day-old baguette,
toasted

1. Warm the oil in a large pot and add the celeriac, potatoes, leek, onions, and shallots. Cook for 10 minutes over medium heat, stirring every once in a while. Add the vegetable stock and bay leaf, season with salt and pepper, and bring to a boil.

2. Reduce heat, then cover and simmer over low heat until the vegetables are tender, 15 to 20 minutes. Add the milk, stir well, and cook for another 5 minutes. Serve, placing a warm toasted baguette slice on top of each bowl.

N.B. THE TRADITIONAL RECIPE CALLS FOR CROUTONS, BREAD PIECES FRIED IN OIL. WE FIND LEFTOVER TOASTED BAGUETTE MUCH LIGHTER AND JUST AS DELICIOUS.

· ·

MIXED VEGETABLE SOUP

Serves 4

1. Warm 1 tablespoon of the oil in a large pot. Sweat the onion, add the leeks, and season with salt and pepper to taste. Add the carrots, potatoes, zucchini, chicken stock, and spinach. Bring to a boil, then cover and simmer for 20 minutes, until all the vegetables are tender.

2. Purée in a food mill and serve with a drizzle of remaining oil and the basil, if using.

INGREDIENTS

2 tablespoons olive oil

1 onion, peeled and chopped

4 leeks, white parts only, sliced

Salt and freshly ground pepper

2 carrots, sliced

1/2 pound potatoes, peeled and coarsely cubed

2 zucchini, diced

1 quart chicken stock

1/2 pound spinach, washed and chopped

2 tablespoons basil chiffonade for garnish (optional)

N.B. IN THE SUMMER, THIS SOUP CAN BE SERVED COLD. REMOVE IT FROM THE REFRIGERATOR 20 MINUTES BEFORE SERVING. ADD A DRIZZLE OF LEMON JUICE AND REPLACE THE BASIL WITH FRESH MINT OR CILANTRO.

SEA SCALLOPS WITH CITRUS FRUIT

Serves 4

Scallops are another shellfish that intimidates some, but they are amazingly simple to make: the key, in fact, is not to do too much to them. While fresh herbs are still around, I love to sear scallops, adding plenty of fresh sage leaves for flavor. In the dead of winter, though, when there is no sage, but lots of scallops, this preparation is a favorite.

INGREDIENTS

16 sea scallops

Zest and juice of ½ grapefruit

Zest and juice of ½ orange

Zest and juice of ½ lemon

1 tablespoon honey

4 cardamom pods

2 tablespoons olive oil

Salt and freshly ground pepper

2 tablespoons unsalted butter, cut into small pieces

Fleur de sel

1. Rinse the scallops and pat dry. Blanch them in boiling water for 1 minute. In a bowl, whisk together the fruit zest and juice, honey, and cardamom pods.

2. Warm a skillet over medium-high heat. Add the oil to the skillet, season the scallops with salt and pepper, and cook them for 2 minutes on each side. Set the scallops aside on a warm plate and cover with foil.

3. In a saucepan, reduce the juice mixture over medium-high heat for 2 minutes, stirring all the while. Reduce the heat and whisk in the butter a few pieces at a time.

4. Plate the scallops and drizzle with sauce. Sprinkle with a few grains of fleur de sel.

SHRIMP AND TUNA SALAD WITH BANANA AND YOGURT

Serves 4

1. In a salad bowl, combine the shrimp and the banana slices with the lemon juice. Add the tuna, almonds, and raisins to the bowl.

2. For the yogurt dressing: Combine the yogurt and heavy cream, mixing well. Add the paprika and dill, and season with pepper.

3. Add the yogurt dressing to the salad bowl and toss gently. Serve chilled.

INGREDIENTS

1 pound shrimp, peeled, deveined, and cooked

2 bananas, sliced into 1/4-inch pieces

2 tablespoons lemon juice

1 8-ounce can of tuna in water

2 ounces sliced almonds

4 ounces golden raisins, steamed for 2 minutes

FOR THE YOGURT DRESSING:

1 cup plain yogurt

1 tablespoon heavy cream (or sour cream)

Dash of paprika

1 tablespoon freshly chopped dill

Freshly ground pepper

STUFFED CORNISH HENS

Serves 4

INGREDIENTS

FOR THE STUFFING:

⅔ cup uncooked brown rice

½ cup mixed nuts (pine nuts, walnut pieces, whole hazelnuts)

2 tablespoons golden raisins

⅓ cup chicken stock

1 tablespoon minced parsley

1 teaspoon dry herbs (chervil and savory or rosemary and thyme)

Salt and freshly ground pepper

2 Cornish hens (or poussins)

Salt and freshly ground pepper

2 tablespoons unsalted butter, melted

3 tablespoons chicken stock

1. For the stuffing: Bring 2 cups water to a boil. Add the rice and cook for 15 minutes. Drain the rice and mix well with the remaining stuffing ingredients. Season stuffing with salt and pepper to taste and refrigerate overnight.

2. Preheat the oven to 475 degrees. Rinse the Cornish hens and dry them inside and out with paper towels and season with salt and pepper to taste. Stuff the birds loosely with the rice mixture and truss. Put the remaining stuffing aside in a small oven-proof dish.

3. Put the hens in a baking dish, brush them with melted butter and season again with the salt and pepper. Bake in the preheated oven for 10 minutes, then baste with the chicken stock. Continue to baste every 10 minutes. After 20 minutes, reduce the temperature to 350 degrees and put the dish of stuffing into the oven. Roast the hens for another 20 minutes. Serve immediately with a tablespoon of stuffing on each side of the hens as garnish.

N.B. THIS, I HAVE FOUND, IS A WONDERFUL VALENTINE'S DAY DINNER. WHILE THE HENS ARE IN THE OVEN YOU HAVE TIME TO CONCOCT A LITTLE DESSERT. *ET VOILÀ*, YOU CAN SIT DOWN FOR A CANDLELIT DINNER.

. . . .

GARLICKY MONKFISH

Serves 4

1. Warm the oil and sauté garlic in a large skillet over medium heat until the garlic is cooked, but not brown. Add the tomato paste and white wine and mix well.

2. Add the monkfish and cook over medium to low heat for 10 minutes on each side. Season with salt and pepper to taste and sprinkle with basil. Serve immediately.

INGREDIENTS

4 tablespoons olive oil

4 teaspoons finely minced garlic

2 tablespoons tomato paste

1 cup white wine

1 pound monkfish

Salt and freshly ground pepper

1/4 cup basil chiffonade

. . . .

SALMON WITH ORANGE *EN PAPILLOTE*

Serves 4

1. Preheat the oven to 350 degrees.

2. In a small saucepan, combine all ingredients for the marinade and season with salt and pepper to taste. Bring to a simmer over medium heat until the marinade is reduced by half. Remove from the heat and set aside. Cut 8 large pieces of parchment paper (or aluminum foil) into squares large enough to cover each fish fillet and leave a 2-inch border all around. Lightly brush 4 squares with olive oil.

INGREDIENTS

FOR THE MARINADE:

1/4 cup orange juice

1 tablespoon lemon juice

1 tablespoon dry vermouth

2 tablespoons soy sauce

1 tablespoon minced ginger

Pinch of sugar

Salt and freshly ground pepper

INGREDIENTS

Olive oil

4 skinless fillets of salmon,
about 4 ounces each

Salt and freshly ground
pepper

3. Put each salmon fillet in the center of an oiled square and drizzle with the marinade. Season with salt and pepper to taste.

4. Place the remaining squares on top of the fillets, and fold up the edges to form packets. Simply double folding each of the four sides is enough to seal each package. Put the *papillotes* on a baking sheet, and bake in the preheated oven for 12 to 15 minutes. Serve with brown rice.

. . . .

CHICKEN TATIN

Serves 6

INGREDIENTS

8 tablespoons olive oil

1 3- to 3½-pound chicken,
cut in pieces

2 tablespoons chopped
shallots

2 cinnamon sticks

3 cardamom pods

1 quart chicken stock

Salt and freshly ground
pepper

1. In a large heavy skillet, warm up 2 tablespoons of oil, and brown the chicken on all sides over medium-high heat. Leaving the chicken in the skillet, lower the heat and add the shallots, cinnamon sticks, cardamom, and chicken stock. Season with salt and pepper to taste. Bring to a boil on high heat. Cover, lower the heat to medium, and simmer for another 30 to 35 minutes.

2. Remove the chicken from the skillet and reserve the stock. When cool enough to

handle, remove the skin and bones and discard.

3. Add 4 tablespoons of oil to a large frying pan and cook the eggplant 5 minutes on each side. Remove and pat dry on paper towels.

4. Mix the turmeric with ½ cup of the reserved stock. In the skillet, warm the remaining 2 tablespoons of oil over medium-high heat, add the rice, and cook until it becomes translucent, about 10 minutes. Remove half of the rice and reserve. Flatten the remaining rice in the skillet and layer ½ the eggplant and all the chicken pieces. Cover with the remaining eggplant and top with the remaining rice. Pour the turmeric-stock mixture over the rice and add 5 cups of the reserved stock. Cover the skillet. Bring to a boil, lower the heat to medium, and cook for about 30 to 35 minutes, or until all the liquid is absorbed. Allow to rest 10 minutes.

5. To serve, use a platter, like a tatin tart, unmold the chicken tatin on the platter. Add the pine nuts, raisins, and a bowl of yogurt as an accompaniment.

INGREDIENTS

2 large eggplants, unpeeled, sliced thinly lengthwise

1 teaspoon turmeric

16 ounces basmati rice

2 ounces pine nuts, toasted

2 tablespoons golden raisins

1 quart yogurt

DUCK BREASTS WITH HONEY GLAZE

Serves 4

Americans rarely cook a whole duck. Today, duck breasts are available in most supermarkets or on the Internet, making a taste of canard *easy and quick. Duck isn't as lean as turkey, but it has less saturated fat than most red meats. Though a rich food, and so not to be overdone, it's very digestible and* moelleux *(soft).*

INGREDIENTS

2 duck breasts (4 *magrets*), about 1½ pounds

4 tablespoons sherry vinegar

4 tablespoons honey

2 tablespoons chicken stock

Salt and freshly ground pepper

1. Sear the breasts in a skillet over medium-high heat, about 3 minutes per side. Set aside.

2. Pour the fat off the skillet and reduce the heat to medium. Add the vinegar and scrape up any bits sticking to the bottom of the pan. Stir in the honey and chicken stock.

3. Cut the duck into ½-inch strips, return to the pan with the sauce, and cook briefly until done, according to taste. Season with salt and pepper to taste, remove, and arrange on plates. Drizzle sauce on top.

N.B. YOU CAN USE A SIMILAR SAUCE WITH PORK OR CHICKEN.

· ·

DUCK BREASTS SWEET AND SOUR

Serves 4

1. To make the sauce: Pour the orange and grapefruit juices in a small saucepan and reduce by half over high heat. Add the honey, vinegar, and pepper, and stir until all the ingredients are well mixed. Add the veal stock. Cook, uncovered, over low heat for 15 minutes. Season with salt to taste and set aside.

2. Peel the pear and apple. Core them and slice thinly. Put the slices in a saucepan with the lemon juice. Add the cinnamon and 1/3 cup water and cook over medium-low heat for 15 minutes. Set aside on a warm plate.

3. Remove the skin from the duck breasts and salt lightly. Warm a nonstick pan over medium heat and cook the breasts for 2 minutes on each side. Cover and continue to cook for 8 minutes.

4. Slice the breasts and arrange them in a fan on each dish. Put the pear and apple compote on the side and pour the sauce over everything.

INGREDIENTS

3 ounces orange juice

3 ounces grapefruit juice

2 tablespoons honey

3 ounces sherry vinegar

1/4 teaspoon pepper

1 cup veal stock

Salt

1 pear

1 apple

Juice of 1 lemon

1/4 teaspoon cinnamon

2 duck breasts (4 *magrets*), about 1 1/2 pounds

COCOTTE DE LÉGUMES (VEGETABLES) CROQUANTS

Serves 4

I discovered this dish in St.-Rémy-de-Provence, the village that inspired van Gogh's Starry Night *vision. One late fall day, the weather went from T-shirt sunny to earmuff frosty overnight. "It hasn't been this cold this early in years," the locals kept saying. After an unexpected numbing two days, I was ready for something to warm my innards. And I am always ready for vegetables. Walking down Boulevard Victor Hugo, meters from where van Gogh painted* Les Paveurs *(1889), I saw Cocotte de Légumes Croquants on the blackboard menu outside the Café des Arts, a bistro-style restaurant and bar. A* cocotte *is a cast-iron covered pot, and just the idea of piping-hot vegetables cooking in one drew me in. The dish was delicious, a heart-warming single course for a wintry day's lunch or as part of dinner.*

INGREDIENTS

4 tablespoons olive oil

2 medium shallots, peeled and cut in half

3 pounds of mixed vegetables (carrots, leeks, haricots verts, fennel, celery, broccoli, squash, and beets), peeled, rinsed, and cut into medium pieces

1 pear, peeled and cut in half

1 apple, peeled and cut in half

Juice of 1 lemon

Salt and freshly ground pepper

1. Put the *cocotte* (or any large heavy-bottomed pot) over medium-low heat. Add the oil and shallots and cook for 2 minutes. Add all the vegetables, fruit, lemon juice, and ½ cup water. Mix, season with salt and pepper to taste, and cover. Cook for 50 minutes, stirring occasionally. Some of the vegetables will still be a bit firm (*al dente*) while others will be *moelleux* (soft).

2. Serve piping hot in a soup bowl or perhaps in individual-sized, warmed *cocottes*.

SHALLOTS *CONFITES EN PAPILLOTE*

Serves 4

A word on shallots. Onions, garlic, shallots, and leeks are all in the same family, but therein lies a world of nuance. For the French, the shallot is "un légume bien de chez nous" *(a vegetable that's very much us) since we have quasi-cornered its production (it grows in Brittany, the Loire, the south and southwest). It wouldn't be French if there weren't different varieties to enjoy, from the strongest, which is called* "grise" *and has thick skin, to the "chicken leg," which is longer, more coppery in color, and more subtle in flavor, to the medium-sized specimen with its mild taste and pinkish color, and finally to the rarest one of all, the small round one. We have recently turned our neighbors in Germany into voracious shallot consumers and are making headway in other countries as well. It's easy to see why: the shallot is low in calories but filled with vitamin C, iron, calcium, selenium, and sulfuric anti-germ components. Besides, it influences and accents a dish's flavor like you wouldn't believe. As the cooks in my family used to say, the shallot adds* "tonus dans vos plats" *(tone). We use it in every way, everywhere: raw and finely minced in salads or with cooked vegetables, grilled meats, or fresh cheese with fresh herbs. Cooked, it completes classic sauces, is great in an omelet or rice dish, and it can be cooked with butter, a pinch of sugar, and a splash of red wine to accompany fish or white meat. When* confites *shallots become a delectable mush— in appearance something like baby food, but in taste something else altogether.*

1. Preheat the oven to 250 degrees.

2. Rub the unpeeled shallots with butter and put them on a large sheet of aluminum foil. Cover with another sheet and fold up all around to seal.

INGREDIENTS

1 pound unpeeled shallots (the long variety is best)

2 tablespoons unsalted butter, at room temperature

3. Cook in the preheated oven for at least an hour. When soft, remove and cut each shallot in half. Serve as a vegetable with a dish like pork roast; the melted shallot flesh is eaten with a spoon.

IN ALSACE, MY GRANDMOTHER WOULD MAKE BIG BATCHES OF THIS DELICIOUS "SHALLOT MEAT." AT LEAST ONCE A WEEK SHE WOULD TAKE IT OUT OF THE FRIDGE BEFORE LUNCH AND THEN SERVE IT AT ROOM TEMPERATURE ON A SLICE OF COUNTRY BREAD INSTEAD OF THE LUNCH CHEESE COURSE. ADD A FEW GRAINS OF COARSE SALT AND SAVOR.

. . . .

BRAISED FENNEL WITH GINGER

Serves 4

I love fennel and don't see it served in restaurants enough or in many recipes for home. Too bad. High in water content, rich in fiber, and oh so flavorful, it gives a zing to any salad or as a vegetable accompaniment to a main course. Healthy and rich in potassium, vitamins C and E, and beta carotene, an antioxidant, fennel can be consumed raw, thinly sliced, or cooked with a bit of olive oil and shallots or garlic. When picking fennel, look for tender green fronds, a sign of freshness, and always favor thick-stem bulbs.

INGREDIENTS

4 fennel bulbs
4 tablespoons olive oil
2 tablespoons finely minced fresh ginger
Pinch of cumin

1. Cut the fennel bulbs in half lengthwise. Chop each half into four pieces.

2. Warm the oil in a saucepan over medium heat. Add the ginger and cook for 10 seconds. Add the cumin and white wine and bring to a boil. Add the fennel pieces and

lemon juice, season with salt and pepper to taste, and simmer for 20 minutes over medium-low heat, until the fennel is softened and flavors are blended. Serve with most fish or white meats.

. . . .

BRAISED CARROTS WITH GINGER

Serves 4

1. Wash the carrots and slice thinly. Toss the carrots with the zest and juice of the orange and lemon, the ginger, onions, and oil, and season with salt and pepper to taste.

2. Warm the butter in a saucepan. When it is melted, add all the ingredients except the cilantro, and cook over medium-low heat for 20 minutes. Add the fresh cilantro and serve.

INGREDIENTS

4 carrots, about 1 pound

Zest and juice of 1 orange

Zest and juice of 1 lemon

2 teaspoons finely minced fresh ginger

2 medium onions, peeled and minced

2 tablespoons olive oil

Salt and freshly ground pepper

2 tablespoons unsalted butter

2 tablespoons minced fresh cilantro

. . . .

In winter, "the wise trees," as William Carlos Williams writes, "stand sleeping in the cold." The wise French woman, however, knows this is not an option, much as the duvet may beckon. Still, lovers of fruit—an indispensable element of the French woman's *bien-être*—will find themselves relatively hard-pressed in winter. Never are the pickings slimmer. I still enjoy apples, pears, and bananas that seem to come greener and greener as the days pass (I've waited for up to two weeks for some bananas in a brown bag to ripen). Here is a time when those of us who live in the northern climes simply can't go it alone with local produce. In the old days we may have got by with preserved fruit in a jar; there is still a place for that. But I can't survive a whole season without fresh fruit. Without nature's sugar for dessert, my sweet tooth would lead me to a surfeit of pastry temptation. Anyway, I would surely struggle not to get fat *sans fruits*. This does not mean I abandon the seasonality principle. There are still fruits I enjoy only in winter, regardless of how much big-time global agribusiness and marketing wants to make them available year-round. It simply means that I enjoy fruits that aren't the most perishable shipped in from places where they are picked in season. The mainstay of my winter fruit fix is fresh citrus, especially from Florida, and for this I go to the source.

One of America's best-kept secrets is oranges and grapefruits fresh from the groves, not from the supermarket. One winter, some years ago, I had to attend an event in Miami. At the breakfast buffet in my hotel, I rather routinely picked a grapefruit half. To my astonishment, I had never tasted a grapefruit that good. Shiny, juicy, miraculous—a half moon on my plate. I kept squeezing it for the last few drops of juice, marveling at its difference from all the other grapefruits I'd ever eaten. Being a French woman, I had been under the impression that I was buying *zee best*. Could it have simply been the mesmerizing effect of sitting on the lovely terrace looking at the water and the sun? When the pleasure was recaptured on each subsequent day, I knew this was no placebo effect. It did not take much trouble to discover that the grapefruits came from Indian River and how simple it was to order them.

Many native New Yorkers, it turned out, already knew about this "tradition" of having fruit shipped from Florida, and I have converted dozens of friends to my winter tactic. At first, they are invariably stunned that for about the same price that supermarkets charge you can have fruit that is so indisputably superior. Anyone can order Florida citrus online or by phone. And having spread the good word, I'm now the lucky recipient of several gift boxes from friends, which furnish my citrus cure every winter. The varieties of fresh oranges are all sensational, and the tangelos, which are in season only a few weeks a year in January, are especially sublime. Serve them on Sunday in place of orange juice or for dessert as an afternoon pick-me-up. (They go deliciously with that other pick-me-up, dark chocolate.) The divine orangey sweetness has, in my experience, been rivaled only by the freshest blood oranges, tasted in Morocco years ago.

ARDÈCHE COFFEE

Serves 4

Ardèche was where my chef-trained Uncle Charles moved when he married Aunt Mireille. It's also chestnut land, and for a coffee lover this simple winter dessert is heavenly.

INGREDIENTS

4 tablespoons mascarpone

1 teaspoon sugar

2 teaspoons glazed chestnuts, crumbled

4 scoops coffee ice cream

2 glazed chestnuts, split in half

4 shots espresso

1. Whip the mascarpone and sugar together and divide it among 4 glass dessert bowls. Sprinkle each with the crumbled chestnuts. Add a scoop of coffee ice cream and place half a chestnut on top. Refrigerate.

2. When ready to serve, pour a very hot espresso over each serving.

N.B. YOU CAN BUY GLAZED CHESTNUTS IN A CHOCOLATE SHOP OR VIA THE INTERNET. AN ALTERNATIVE IS AMARETTO COOKIES FOUND IN ITALIAN BAKERIES OR SPECIALTY SHOPS.

· ·

BANANA MOUSSE

Serves 4

1. Mash the bananas with the lemon and orange juice. Add the honey and vanilla extract and mix well. Add the yogurt and mix well.

2. In a separate bowl, beat the egg whites until they are stiff, and fold them gently into the banana mixture. Refrigerate for at least 1 hour before serving.

INGREDIENTS

3 very ripe bananas, peeled

Juice of 2 lemons

Juice of 3 oranges

2 tablespoons honey

1 teaspoon vanilla extract

1 cup yogurt

3 egg whites

. . . .

COFFEE MOUSSE

Serves 6

1. Beat the egg whites with the salt until very firm and set aside. Whip the heavy cream with sugar. Slowly incorporate the espresso into the whipped cream. Carefully fold the espresso cream into the egg whites.

2. Spoon the coffee mousse into 6 bowls or cups and refrigerate for at least 1 hour before serving.

INGREDIENTS

4 egg whites

Pinch of salt

1 cup heavy cream

⅔ cup sugar

4 tablespoons strong espresso, chilled

N.B. I LOVE TO SERVE THIS MOUSSE AFTER DINNER (INSTEAD OF OFFERING COFFEE) WITH FRESH BABY MADELEINES.

. . . .

HOT CHOCOLATE SOUFFLÉ

Serves 6

INGREDIENTS

½ cup milk (regular or 2 percent)

½ cup unsweetened Dutch cocoa powder

⅓ cup sugar, plus extra for dusting soufflé mold

4 eggs, at room temperature, separated

2 tablespoons unsalted butter, at room temperature, plus extra for buttering soufflé mold

Pinch of salt

1. Preheat the oven to 350 degrees. Prepare a 1-quart soufflé mold by lightly buttering it, dusting the insides with sugar, and tapping out the excess. Place the mold in the refrigerator.

2. Pour the milk, cocoa powder, and sugar into a heavy saucepan and stir to combine. Bring to a boil over moderate heat, stirring constantly. Reduce the heat and cook, still stirring, until the mixture thickens, about 10 minutes. Transfer to a bowl and cool slightly.

3. Stir the egg yolks into the warm chocolate mixture. Stir in the butter.

4. In a separate bowl, beat the egg whites until they reach soft peaks. Add the salt and beat until stiff. Whisk half of the egg whites mixture into the chocolate mixture. Fold in the remaining egg whites gently with a spatula. Pour the mixture into the soufflé mold and smooth the top.

5. Bake on the lower-middle shelf of the preheated oven until puffy and brown, about 18 minutes, which will give you a soft center. Serve at once with whipped cream.

MANGO CARPACCIO WITH CINNAMON

Serves 4

1. Put the sugar in a small saucepan with the lemon juice, 1 mint leaf, and 2 tablespoons water. Bring to a boil and remove from the heat. Stir until the sugar is well dissolved. Remove the mint leaf and add the cinnamon. Let cool.

2. Cut the mangoes into halves, running a sharp knife around the pits to detach. Peel and slice thinly. Arrange the slices on 4 serving dishes and drizzle with the sugar syrup. Cover and refrigerate for 15 minutes. Decorate with mint leaves when ready to serve.

INGREDIENTS

2 tablespoons sugar

Juice of 1 lemon

Fresh mint leaves

½ teaspoon cinnamon

2 ripe mangoes

. . . .

A final word on surviving those fruitless months: consider the pomegranate. It's a loaded proposition. The consumption of the seeds of this fruit cultivated since ancient times constituted Persephone's ill-fated prenup. (With such luck as hers, to say nothing of Eve's travails on account of eating an apple, or whatever it was, it is small wonder the entire female gender has not forsworn fruit.) Looking beyond mythic admonitions, however, the modern French woman loves to toss a handful of sweet juicy pomegranate seeds in a winter salad. Lately, the unrivaled heart-health benefits of pomegranates have become very well known—they are loaded with polyphenols, even more so than red wine. As for me, I am captivated by their flavor. Pried from a husk that is utterly inedible, they are a comforting reminder that Persephone's sojourn in the underworld, and ours in winter, is not eternal or even so terrible.

The other precious token of warmer times and climes—without which I'd find winter unbearable—is flowers. In regions where the temperature drops to freezing, the container-plant gardener starts looking inward: well, indoors at least. There's a great tradition of this in France, from the Court of Versailles to the Luxembourg Garden of today where the palaces all had orangeries—large pavilions where the orange, palm, and other fragile potted (in very large containers, indeed) plants were moved indoors to winter. While Edward and I don't have anything like the Sun King's potted fruit trees, one thing we do have is a nice pot with a chest-high jasmine plant that we bring indoors. It seems to enjoy its winter residence, rewarding our solicitude by flowering several times a season indoors and filling our home with a divine aroma.

The year-end holidays have their own indoor plant and flower traditions that add some color and life to an already colorful period. Poinsettias can't be denied their brightness, but are far from my favorites. We are, however, lovers of Christmas trees and wreaths. The notion of the evergreen (the pomegranate is one, too, by the way) is a lovely little defiance of the implacable rhythm of seasonality by which we all live. And the scent is so soothing.

During the holidays and afterward, cut flowers and flower centerpieces seem to find their way into our home and the homes we visit. Admittedly they represent an extravagance at this time of year, but if you make simple, thoughtful choices, and take care to extend their lives by cutting stems and changing water, these blooms do qualify as affordable luxuries.

January through March is a special interval for the year in flowers. That's orchid season. The variety, availability, and beauty of these glorious container flowers are a godsend of color and vitality in winter, when it's a great comfort to be welcomed home by one after work. They are not cheap, and indeed, they were once emblems of the extravagance and care-free obsessions of the rich. But prices have remained stable in recent years, thanks to better distribution and supply. In any case, their long bloom time makes them cost-effective. If you buy an orchid with only a few open flowers and many buds, it will continue to flower for anywhere from six weeks to three months. When the plant is past blooming, the leaves are attractive enough to serve as a green plant for a while if you snip off the dead flower stalk. We can usually get through the winter replacing orchid plants only once, and we're never without a bloom. When we start to get really itchy for spring, we grow some forced bulbs in pots indoors—grape and regular hyacinths, tulips, daffodils, paperwhites. There is something about watching a flower grow day by day, from bud to blossom, that is pleasurable and fulfilling, renewing one's faith in renewal, just when the cold seems it will never end.

• A Week's Menu for Winter •

<table>
<tr><td>

Breakfast
2 prunes
2 scrambled eggs
1 slice whole wheat bread,
    toasted and buttered
Coffee or tea

Lunch
1 cup vegetable soup
½ cup yogurt
1 grapefruit
Noncaloric beverage

Dinner
Mustard Rabbit (*Lapin*) *en*
    Papillote (page 246)
Potato-Olive Ragout
    (page 156)
Green salad
1 tangerine
1 glass white or red wine

</td><td>

Breakfast
1 ounce cheese
½ cup fruit compote
1 slice sourdough bread,
    toasted and buttered
Coffee or tea

Lunch
Chicken breast with tarragon
½ cup green vegetables
½ cup cottage cheese
4 dried apricots
Noncaloric beverage

Dinner
Spaghetti carbonara
½ cup mushrooms
½ cup carrots
Green salad
Spiced Apples (page 174)
1 glass red wine

</td></tr>
</table>

• A Week's Menu for Winter •

Breakfast
1 slice boiled ham
½ cup cream of wheat
½ cup milk
½ teaspoon honey
1 slice seven-grain bread,
    toasted and buttered
Coffee or tea

Lunch
Shrimp or tuna salad
½ bagel
2 clementines
Noncaloric beverage

Dinner
Salmon with Orange *en
    Papillote* (page 217)
½ cup spinach
3 ounces potatoes
Pears with Chocolate and
    Pepper (page 175)
1 glass red wine

Breakfast
½ grapefruit
½ cup yogurt with 3 table-
    spoons bran flakes
1 slice multigrain bread,
    toasted and buttered
Coffee or tea

Lunch
1 cup Lentil Soup
    (page 160)
1 cup salad
2 kiwis
1 square chocolate
Noncaloric beverage

Dinner
Duck Breasts with Honey
    Glaze (page 220)
Sautéed fennel
½ cup yogurt
1 apple
1 glass red wine

• A Week's Menu for Winter •

Breakfast
½ cup orange juice or
   1 orange
1 soft-boiled egg
1 slice whole wheat bread,
   toasted and buttered
Coffee or tea

Lunch
Turkey sandwich
1 cup green salad
1 pear
Noncaloric beverage

Dinner
Sea Scallops with Citrus
   Fruit (page 214)
½ cup brown rice
1 banana flambée
1 glass Champagne or
   sparkling wine

Breakfast
1 slice prosciutto
½ cup Grandma Louise's
   Oatmeal with Grated
   Apple (www
   .mireilleguiliano.com)
½ cup milk
½ English muffin, toasted
   and buttered
Coffee or tea

Lunch
Salad of endives with ham
1 slice country bread
1 papaya
Noncaloric beverage

Dinner
Stuffed Cornish Hens
   (page 216)
½ cup green vegetables
1 slice carrot-ginger cake
1 glass red wine

• A Week's Menu for Winter •

Breakfast
1 ounce cheese
2 pancakes with 2 table-
    spoons maple syrup
½ cup yogurt
Coffee or tea

Lunch (main meal)
6 oysters
Garlicky Monkfish
    (page 217)
½ cup uncooked green
    vegetables
1 large sweet potato
Banana Mousse (page 229)
1 glass Champagne or
    white wine

Dinner
1 cup Mixed Vegetable Soup
    (page 213)
1 slice bread
½ cup yogurt
½ grapefruit

ENTR'ACTE: THE FRENCH EAT *WHAT*?

When I was an exchange student outside Boston, some of my classmates and their parents called me "Frenchy." It was a lot easier to remember and pronounce than "Mireille" [meer-RAY], and as they said it with affection I was fine with it. Sometimes, though, I was also referred to as "Froggie" or "our Frog friend, Mireille." It seemed a little weird and it honestly took another twenty years before I made the connection. Other people call the French "Frogs" because, well, we eat frogs, a habit that seems mostly alien and, to some Americans, almost beyond belief. I can just imagine an earlier era when this custom became common knowledge in America: the GIs coming back from World War II saying, "And they eat frogs!" *Et voilà. Dis-moi ce que tu manges, et je te dirai ce que tu es.* (Tell me what you eat, and I'll tell you what you are. Brillat-Savarin was right about most things.)

Well, I do love to eat frogs (we eat just the legs), as do lots of French people. They are delicious simply sautéed in oil, butter, and garlic with some parsley. And we eat snails and fattened goose livers and pigeons and rabbits and sorrel and dandelions, plus a lot more delicious creatures, animal body parts, and plants. Every culture and cuisine has its signifiers.

To many people elsewhere, eating frogs may still be like eating from another planet. You have to remember that American openness to foreign cuisine is still fairly recent, mostly introduced by immigrants in the twentieth century. The French, however, were not a major immigrant group during those great waves.

For a generation of Americans able to take advantage of the democratization of air travel, however, there is no need to depend on hearsay: direct observation of how the French eat is more common. And now many, especially those who have heard the gospel of taste, are more accepting of our weirder edibles, knowing that the best food and wine is that most intimately connected with *le terroir*—the land that gave rise to it. And what could be closer to the muddy earth than a frog? There are many other foodstuffs emblematic of foreign gastronomies that still give some Americans the willies, even as people have been taking cultivated pleasure in these foods for centuries. This interlude is dedicated to a bit of special pleading for a few of the odder seeming foods of the French, things that I left out of the seasonal program, recognizing that you have to walk before you can run. I don't expect you to race out and make all these things. The French woman's lifestyle requires only that you maintain your equilibrium by appreciating the best that can be found in your locale. Still, the things I describe here are familiar elements of French fare, and those who are determined enough can find them. The hope is that you understand at least how one woman's "totally gross" might be another's *"très délicieux."* Anyway, no French woman should be closed to a new experience *en principe.*

When I was growing up, we often had frogs for Sunday supper courtesy of Monsieur Barbier, a large man with a boyishly pink face who was *Mamie*'s supplier of fresh eggs, cheese, and poultry. He'd show up every Saturday, his small truck full of super-fresh food he had collected from farmers in his village and the surrounding area. During frog season, summer and fall, when he was able to collect enough to supply us, his "special customers," he'd call ahead saying he'd be late. As evening arrived, he'd appear with a basket covered with burlap. It set us salivating. The designation "special customers" was probably his way of letting us know he was favoring us with something in relatively limited supply. His way of marketing his customer service. Anyhow, we liked it.

Little did I know, though, that Monsieur Barbier was doing the "dirty work" himself: catching the slippery creatures and dressing them. For me, the mystery was how he managed to obtain only the parts we ate, the legs. What he delivered under the burlap in his *panier* didn't quite fit with La Fontaine's fable or the princes disguised as frogs in my children's books. My father saw the sense in sparing me such life lessons as how frogs become frogs' legs or how the bunnies I played with would be skinned and cleaned for *ragoût de lapin.* Somehow he always managed to evade my inquisitiveness. And to this day I'm not quite sure how it's done. On the rare occasion when I have a dish of frogs' legs before me (as at New York's *grande dame* La Grenouille, The Frog, an apt enough name for a French restaurant) my mind is fixed only on savoring the succulent little bundles without a thought to the practical considerations. But I do always think of dear Monsieur Barbier... *le porteur de grenouilles* (the frog bearer), with his cheerful face. I like to think that by continuing to indulge this pleasure so many years on, I am honoring his frog-catching efforts.

I will not provide more of a recipe for frogs' legs than the sautée I mentioned above, which works well with the legs plain or breaded. The challenge is not in cooking them, but in finding them. They are not readily available in the United States, although in Florida, Georgia, and Northern California I have found traditions of serving frogs and good purveyors.

What I will tell you, however, is where you can enjoy the greatest frog dish on earth. It is in Alsace, at the three-star Michelin restaurant Buerehiesel in Strasbourg. The *schnieder-späetle* (a kind of noodle) and frogs' legs *poêlées* with chervil is something any food lover should hope to experience at least once. At Beurehiesel, the culinary alchemists sauté the little drumsticks with oil, butter, parsley, and probably a few other secret ingredients. You pick up the tiny legs with your fingers and the thighs melt in your mouth, exploding with flavor. Why are their frogs so great? The cooking, ambience, and service, sure, but the restaurant seems to have an exemplary purveyor for special frogs fed some fare not to be found in any old pond. (If you are what you eat—and you are—the better or distinctively good your food is fed, the better you and it will be, so think what your food eats is who you are.) In any case, we have been mightily tempted to order a second helping, in defiance of my golden rule of pleasures in moderation. (Then again, everyone has her indulgences—why not frogs?) It is worth mentioning that the famed wine guru Robert Parker is likewise nuts about this dish at Buerehiesel and has indeed confessed to ordering seconds. His wine pairing, however, and whether perhaps he didn't order them for dessert must remain a matter of speculation.

PIGEON

Readers of *French Women Don't Get Fat* will recall my father's comment when he collected me off the boat twenty-plus pounds heavier after my year in America: *"Tu ressembles à un sac de patates"* (You look like a sack of potatoes). Don't judge: he had many endearing qualities, though tact was not among them. He was generally fair but no flatterer, to be sure, and he always spoke his mind. So when he said something nice, however belatedly, you knew he meant it. It took a year, well after I had regained my former shape thanks to Dr. Miracle, before my father told me *"Tu es à nouveau mon p'tit pigeon voyageur"* (You are again my little homing pigeon). The compliment makes particular sense in my family context.

In addition to his gardening and beekeeping, my father had a third hobby as a member of a *société de pigeons voyageurs* (a club devoted to homing pigeons). We had about sixty birds in a special house, *le pigeonnier,* across a courtyard behind our house. Twice a day he'd go visit and feed them a special mix of organic grains he'd prepared as well as refill their water and make sure their quarters were clean. No matter how tired he was after work, his *p'tits pigeons* got their TLC.

I was allowed, albeit only in his company, to see the tiny eggs, the baby pigeons, the growing ones. He would speak to them, looking each one over to see whether it was ready for its first flight. Some of them would never earn his respect, never make the cut, and he'd joke that they would become *les bâtards* (city pigeons): he meant the fat, shapeless, graceless, lazy birds to be found in cities all over the world; they just eat all day from whatever junk the locals or visitors feed them, and often they grow diseased. Fairly or not, my father had little sympathy for creatures that let themselves go. Living well and in balance was the way to earn his admiration.

To be a *pigeon voyageur* you had to be in shape, lean and nice-looking. A *pigeon voyageur* stood up tall, its plumage neat, its eyes clear and sharp, its moves clean and "in the zone." The difference with the city pigeons was enormous. Early this spring, I was reminded of his distinction as I watched people shuffling out of a movie theater on Broadway. To my sadness I saw many women and men lumbering heftily, grazing without a thought, looking for all the world like city pigeons.

A few times as a child I was allowed to watch the birds make love and later lay eggs and take care of their hatchlings. There was a strange beauty in their simple instinctive life. Flying long distances kept them in shape and they could compete for a few years before settling down to bring up a new generation of healthy pigeons. A life of wholesome food, healthful exertion, close to and in sync with the *terroir.*

My father prized his pigeons, but he did not sentimentalize them. He was breeding birds with two purposes: one was the enjoyment of a young *pigeon rôti* (roast pigeon, which today appears more typically as "squab" on the menus of good restaurants). Served with fresh spring peas it is one of the simplest and most delicious meals I have ever had. It was a treat we would enjoy for just a few Sundays each spring, always with great anticipation. Eating the roast pigeon with its little bones meant using your fingers, so this dish was my first exposure to the *rince-doigts,* or finger bowl, which was really more a practical necessity for a simple meal than a formal dining affectation.

Of course, only a few pigeons would be roasted, as I say. My father's real love was the race. From late spring to early summer, he would select the "cream of the flock" for competition, as each member of the pigeon society would do. The pigeons would be sent by train to, let's say, Brest, Biarritz, or Barcelona, where they would rest overnight before being released to fly back home. On Sunday afternoons Dad was often fairly consumed with impatience while waiting for them. Once a bird crossed the threshold of the *pigeonnier* an alarm would click, and my father would hasten to remove the little silver ring around its foot, which he would insert into a special clock that officially registered the exact arrival time. At the end of the season, after all the society pigeons had made the trip home from a dozen cities across Europe and nearby, the winners were announced. My father, or Justin, as his fellows in the *société* knew him, was always in the top three. It was a great source of pride, as were those trophies I remember, with silver or gold pigeons atop them. It seems odd to some, this intense relation my father had with these birds, some of which we ate. In fact it was quite natural: he loved them as pigeons, not as people, and as kept pigeons they were meant for food or flight.

PIGEON RÔTI

Serves 4

1. Warm a *cocotte* over medium heat, then add the oil, butter, shallots, tomatoes, and bacon. Cook a few minutes over medium heat. Add the pigeons. Season with salt and pepper to taste.

2. Cover and cook at low heat for 1½ hours. Uncover for the last 10 minutes. You can serve with fresh peas added to the *cocotte* during the final 10 minutes of cooking. Sprinkle with fresh chopped parsley and serve.

INGREDIENTS

2 tablespoons olive oil

1 tablespoon unsalted butter

2 shallots, peeled and halved

4 small-medium tomatoes, quartered

1 small piece of bacon (about 2 ounces)

4 pigeons (squabs)

Salt and freshly ground pepper

Chopped parsley

. . . .

RABBIT

Europeans routinely eat rabbit. They are, as everyone knows, prolific little animals, and in the old days a peasant could always catch one even when he did not have a chicken to put into his pot. (It was, by the way, Henry IV, the sixteenth-century French king, who made the chicken-in-every-pot promise, long before it became an American campaign pledge.) Cowboys, as we can observe in Westerns, were routinely shooting rabbits for dinner out on the range. It was less a delicacy than a matter of survival. Today, really since the dawn of animation, Americans have given rabbits way too much personality and are skittish about eating Bugs Bunny.

Most gardeners who have lost a crop to rabbits, however, have no qualms about settling the score via a fricassée.

Early in my marriage, we hosted a dinner party for some of Edward's friends. I thought I would do something special and went to Little Italy in Manhattan to buy fresh killed *coniglio*. (One thing about New York, if it is grown, caught, or manufactured, you can buy it . . . and just about anywhere people hunt you are bound to be able to score some rabbit.) While the stew was in the pot, Edward, just informed of the surprise I had planned, speculated that the fare might pose a problem for some of the guests, one woman in particular. The French woman's art of useful deception to the rescue: plate in the kitchen, serve in the dining room, and call it a French chicken *chasseur*. I'm pretty militant about truth in advertising, so this was a very rare exception. Fortunately no one caught on and everyone loved it. To this day, I am sure a couple of those guests would swear they have never eaten rabbit.

Rabbit, like turkey, is a lean meat, low in calories and easy to prepare. Mustard, honey, and prunes are some of the classic preparations.

MUSTARD RABBIT (*LAPIN*) *EN PAPILLOTE*

Serves 4

INGREDIENTS

4 pieces of rabbit (legs or loins)

4 tablespoons Meaux mustard

1. Preheat the oven to 375 degrees.

2. Coat each rabbit piece with a tablespoon of mustard. Cut 8 squares of parchment paper (or aluminum foil) large enough to hold a piece of rabbit and leave a 2-inch

border all around. Lightly brush 4 squares of paper with olive oil. Put a bay leaf in the center of a square, then season with salt and pepper to taste; top with a piece of rabbit and a tablespoon of port wine, then season again; and add a sprig of thyme and a sprig of rosemary.

INGREDIENTS

1 tablespoon olive oil

4 bay leaves

Salt and freshly ground pepper

4 tablespoons port wine

4 sprigs thyme

4 sprigs rosemary

3. Place the remaining parchment squares on top of the rabbit pieces and fold up the edges to form packets. Simply double folding each of the four sides is enough to seal each packet. Put the *papillotes* on a baking sheet and bake in the preheated oven for 45 minutes.

4. Serve by setting each *papillote* on a plate.

N.B. RED OR WHITE WINE CAN BE SUBSTITUTED FOR PORT.

. . . .

RABBIT WITH GRAPES AND WILD MUSHROOMS

Serves 4

Aunt Annie's husband, Robert, was an avid mushroom picker, and in the fall he'd come home with baskets full of an amazing variety of wild cham-pignons. With these pickings and some sweet green table grapes, Aunt Annie would whip up her famous rabbit dish for her two favorite nieces, Claudine and me. She'd announce with a wry smirk that "le chaud lapin" (literally, hot rabbit) was served. It wasn't until years later that Claudine and I got the joke; she was teasing her adoring husband with the slang expression for "womanizer." But I know Robert was faithful to Aunt Annie, and the mushrooms.

INGREDIENTS

3 tablespoons olive oil

1 rabbit cut into 6 pieces

1½ pounds mushrooms, cleaned and sliced (a trio of cèpes, "pleurotes," and chanterelles works wonders)

2 cloves garlic, peeled and minced

3 tablespoons chopped parsley

Salt and freshly ground pepper

2 shallots, minced

3 ounces white wine (approximately 6 tablespoons)

12 ounces chicken stock

3 tablespoons sour cream

1 cup halved green seedless grapes

A handful of chives

1. Warm 2 tablespoons of the oil in a heavy skillet over medium-high heat and sauté the rabbit pieces until they are nicely browned. Remove the rabbit to a side dish while you prepare the mushrooms.

2. In the same skillet sauté the mushrooms and garlic in the remaining tablespoon of oil over medium heat. Add the parsley, season with salt and pepper to taste, and stir. Remove from the skillet and set aside.

3. Put the rabbit pieces back in the skillet along with the shallots and wine. Bring to a simmer and cook for 3 to 5 minutes. Add the stock, season with salt and pepper to taste, cover, and continue simmering 20 minutes, until the rabbit is cooked.

4. Remove the rabbit to a warm plate. Raise the heat and add the mushrooms to cooking liquid. Cook for 5 minutes, then add the sour cream, grapes, and rabbit. Mix and serve, decorating with chives.

N.B. RICE, POTATOES, OR SOME TAGLIATELLE ARE THE PERFECT ACCOMPANIMENT TO THIS DISH.

· ·

ENTR'ACTE

RABBIT LOINS WITH HAZELNUTS

Serves 4

This was another fall/winter dish made by my relatives in the South of France. It's easy and quick; hazelnuts and spices give the dish an unusual touch.

1. Season the rabbit pieces with salt and pepper to taste. Break the eggs on a dinner plate and beat them with a fork. Mix the hazelnuts, four-spice powder, and curry on another dinner plate. Dip the rabbit pieces into the egg mixture, then into the hazelnut-spice mixture.

2. Melt the butter in a skillet; brown the rabbit pieces for 7 to 10 minutes on each side over medium-high heat. Set aside to rest for 5 minutes.

3. Meanwhile, mix the oil and vinegar in a bowl. Season with salt and pepper to taste and toss with the mâche. Serve the salad with the warm rabbit pieces.

INGREDIENTS

4 rabbit loins

Salt and freshly ground pepper

2 eggs

4 ounces hazelnuts, chopped

2 tablespoons four-spice powder

1 teaspoon curry powder

2 tablespoons unsalted butter

2 tablespoons olive oil

1 teaspoon sherry vinegar

1 pound mâche, washed

. . . .

CALF'S LIVER

Say *liver* and you get a funny look from most Americans. It has associations of iron deficiency (children fighting spoonfuls of cod-liver oil). Hannibal Lecter infamously consumed the liver of one of his victims "with fava beans and a nice Chianti" (not a bad pairing).

On the other hand, when offered *foie gras* (French for a *fat liver*), whether from a duck or goose, cold (*en terrine*) or warm, cosmopolitan Americans seem to love it. You can now order it at many restaurants here and across the world. Popularity has created a backlash among the advocates of cruelty-free food who decry the treatment of geese force-fed to fatten their livers. This discontent is perhaps the inevitable result of goose *foie gras*'s having become a commodity. Most liver, however, is simply a by-product of obtaining meat, whether of a chicken or a calf. In America, relatively little of this organ (or any other organs) gets consumed, but in Europe liver is a revered gastronomic tradition. Near our apartment in Paris, a little Italian restaurant named Marco Polo is my regular dispensary for calf's liver Venetian style.

When I grew up, goose liver was reserved for the holiday season, Christmas and New Year's Eve, and occasionally for a very special treat during the year. But Mother was very keen on children eating their slice of calf's liver once a week. It was inexpensive, easy to prepare, and full of nutrients. It is an acquired taste, even for French kids. One of her reliable tricks was to serve it with haricots verts and endives, both of which we loved. Yvette, our *nounou* (nanny), used to call it *le mystère vert veau* (the mystery green calf) making us believe it was veal.

Liver is an excellent food, not lean, but rich in protein and an excellent source of iron for those who are deficient (as a surprising number of young women are). As it is the part of the calf (or of any creature that has one) responsible for the detoxification of the blood, take care in buying it. If possible, the source should be grass-fed and hormone-free.

CALF'S LIVER WITH GREENS

Serves 4

INGREDIENTS

1 pound haricots verts

½ pound endives, cleaned well

1 shallot, minced

5 tablespoons olive oil

1 tablespoon sherry vinegar

1 teaspoon Meaux mustard

Salt and freshly ground pepper

4 slices calf's liver, 3 to 4 ounces each

2 tablespoons flour

1. Bring a saucepan of lightly salted water to a boil. Add the haricots verts and boil for 5 to 7 minutes, until tender. Drain and set aside.

2. Cut the endives into 1-inch slices and set aside.

3. In a bowl, whisk the shallot, 3 tablespoons of the oil, vinegar, mustard, and season with salt and pepper to taste. Add the beans and toss well.

4. Season the calf's liver with salt and pepper and dust lightly with the flour, tapping off any excess. Warm the remaining 2 tablespoons of oil in a large skillet and cook the calf's liver over medium heat, 3 to 4 minutes on each side, until they are golden.

5. Add the endives to the beans and toss well. Serve the liver with the salad (if you have children, cut the liver into small pieces, add it to the salad, and serve in a salad or soup bowl).

In American slang, people sometimes refer to money as lettuce. In French it's sorrel: *avoir de l'oseille* (to have sorrel) is a colloquial way of saying "to be rich." For me, however, the word has a strictly literal connotation: I love this green of distinctively acidic yet slightly bitter taste, similar to but tangier than spinach. I didn't care for it at first, but since it grew like a weed in my father's garden, my mother found ways of slipping it into dishes, and it has become a cherished taste. Sorrel is in season from May to October; though best when fresh, it can be bought in a jar for use year-round. I do wish it were more widely appreciated in America. It originates in North Asia but is greatly enjoyed in France, where it is used mostly in omelets, as a great accompaniment to fish (particularly salmon and monkfish), as well as chicken and veal. It's also delicious in bean or lentil soups.

SALMON WITH SORREL

Serves 4

INGREDIENTS

4 cups sorrel
1 tablespoon olive oil
1 tablespoon unsalted butter
Salt and freshly ground pepper

1. Wash the sorrel and remove the stems and center vein of the leaf. Dry in a salad spinner.

2. Warm the oil and butter in a skillet over medium-low heat. Add the sorrel leaves, seasoning with salt and pepper to taste, and turning them over with a wooden

spoon until they attain an almost melted, purée-like consistency. Cook over low heat until all the water has evaporated, about 5 minutes.

3. Serve as a side dish to the salmon fillets with some boiled new potatoes.

INGREDIENTS

4 pieces wild salmon, 4 ounces each, cooked *à l'Unilatéral* (see www .mireilleguiliano.com)

. . . .

CHICKEN BREASTS WITH SORREL SAUCE

Serves 4

1. To make the stuffing, combine 2 cups of the sorrel, 2 tablespoons of the shallots, 1 tablespoon of the oil, and season with salt and pepper to taste.

2. Make a pocket for the stuffing by loosening the skin from one side of each chicken breast, leaving it attached on the other side as much as possible. Insert stuffing. Season with salt and pepper to taste.

3. Warm the remaining 3 tablespoons of oil over medium heat in a large skillet. Arrange the breasts skin side down and cook until nicely browned, about 10 minutes. Then turn the chicken over and continue to cook for 8 to 10 minutes more. Remove the chicken to a warm platter and cover with foil while making the sauce.

INGREDIENTS

4 cups sorrel, washed and dried

3 tablespoons minced shallots

4 tablespoons olive oil

Salt and freshly ground pepper

4 boneless, skin-on chicken breasts

INGREDIENTS

¼ cup white wine

¼ cup heavy cream

2 tablespoons unsalted butter, cut into small pieces

4. Keep about 1 tablespoon of the drippings from the skillet. Add the remaining 1 tablespoon of the shallots and sauté for a minute or two. Add the white wine and stir to deglaze the skillet. Cook until the wine is reduced and syrupy-looking, about 3 minutes. Add the remaining 2 cups of sorrel. Cook and stir until the sorrel is wilted, about 1 minute. Add 1 cup of water. Bring to a simmer and cook about 5 minutes.

5. Add the heavy cream to the sorrel sauce and season with salt and pepper to taste. Pour the sauce into a blender and purée. Return the purée to the skillet, over medium-low heat, and add the butter a little at a time, until the sauce is thickened and shiny.

6. Slice the chicken breasts on the diagonal and spoon the sorrel sauce over them. Serve with fingerling potatoes or brown rice.

. . . .

SCRAMBLED EGGS WITH SORREL

Serves 4

1. Rinse and dry the sorrel. Chop coarsely. Warm a skillet over medium heat. Add the oil and butter. Sweat the shallots for a minute or two. Add the sorrel and stir to melt it.

2. Beat the eggs, and season with salt and pepper to taste. Pour the eggs over the sorrel and keep stirring until the eggs are cooked. Serve on a slice of brioche.

INGREDIENTS

4 cups sorrel

1 tablespoon olive oil

1 tablespoon unsalted butter

2 shallots, minced

9 eggs

Salt and freshly ground pepper

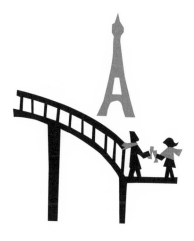

6

WINE IS FOOD

Twenty-five years in the wine business, and I am still embar-
rassed by how much I don't know. Usually, it's no big deal. As
Socrates once said: the more you know the less you know. So,
forget about any insecurity you may have. There's always
more to learn, but you can easily learn enough. The ultimate
reality is simple: given a couple of hours and a couple of bottles, anyone can start enjoying wine.

Sure, there is always a greater subtlety of taste to aspire
to, always more to say—and professional tasters and wine
writers work at doing just that, challenged as they are by the
limits of language to convey the experience of a particular
wine. Ironically, these critics are concerned with describing
the experience for others. Fortunately, as French women we

need describe it only for ourselves. And if we get good enough at it, a relationship with wine can bloom, giving us no end of individual memories by which we can mark our days. The attentive palate is always learning, always assimilating new sensations.

In this sense, I begin with the observation that wine is food. Of course, many others say so, quite correctly, on the basis that wine has nutrients, and let's not forget calories— though a four- to six-ounce glass has no more than a piece of bread or fruit. But if the French woman's secret is pleasure, and the secret of pleasure is taste, the real magic of wine as food is this: nothing else we consume has so much potential for intensity and variety of taste experience. This is so not merely in wine's own right but in the way it complements the tastes of other things we enjoy, as it is meant to do.

Wine isn't seasonal in the way of other foods whose enjoyment we derive from the cyclical receding and renewal of the same pleasures. With wine, we never know exactly what the experience will be, no matter what we've read or heard. Wine, a "living" thing, keeps changing in the bottle as it ages. Nor is there a correct time of year to savor this or that wine— even if some reds may seem too "big" *en principe* for a hot summer's day or if the Beaujolais Nouveau seems interesting to us only when it has just arrived. I drink wine practically every day, and take it from me: most wine can be drunk any time— especially Champagne.

Wine has a different relation to the seasons, one surprisingly like our own. Even with the strictest requirements of *appellations contrôlées* (exacting standards as to composition and production for this to be called Bordeaux or that Rhône), successive vintages are never the same wine. Wine "grows" seasonally like other foods, starting with the grape-growing cycle, which is subject to the vagaries of nature each year. That's why vintners and drinkers began keeping track of years, and distinguishing them. But such statistical zeal, rather like that of American baseball fans, hardly matters to a basic mindful enjoyment. Great enjoyment doesn't necessarily mean "great" vintages, though those experiences can be among the most rewarding, as well as the most costly. Let's just say that each occasion—even of the same wine—forms its own impressions and memories. And if we can learn to pay more thoughtful attention, not only do the experiences feel fuller as we are having them, but they furnish us with another framework in which to make sense of time and make our years seem fuller as well.

The memory of some bottles can stay with you for life. While the wine doesn't have to be old and rare, a great old bottle can be like a time capsule, capturing in its flavors and aromas the time and place of its creation. Veuve Clicquot's 1955 has long been such a mystical vintage for me. Around the time of my twentieth anniversary of working at Clicquot, I could vividly recall the two times I'd tasted it—both occasions strictly in the line of duty, of course. The first time was in Reims at a very formal tasting in the Veuve Clicquot cellars with our superb cellar master, Jacques Peters, and many "wine experts" on hand. That first taste of the 1955 was a revelation, truly an experience of the classical refinement that makes Champagne the king of wines (and the wine of kings). I was unexpectedly transported to those Sunday mornings when, waking to the smell of my mother's brioche in the oven,

I'd be propelled out of bed by the lure of that first bite. I realized the wine was inciting fantasies of what perfect food I could have with it, though in that setting only thin slices of baguette or crackers were to be had. The second occasion, some years later, was a lunch at Veuve Clicquot's mansion we hosted for some very important guests. The 1955 was one of the wines on the menu, and again it was an epiphany: both uncannily recognizable and yet different somehow from the earlier sensation as I recalled it.

But *jamais deux sans trois:* never twice if not thrice, as the French say. In the fall of 1999 Jacques asked me very offhandedly where I would be celebrating the last day of the century. Paris, I said, but very quietly at home; we had long resolved to evade the Y2K mania. "Oh perfect," he said. "I will send you a magnum of '55. We only have a few left in the cellar, and I can't think of anyone who would enjoy it more." You can't put a price on friendship! When I announced this at home it was like Christmas in October. Edward and I immediately realized our moral obligation to invite a few of our close friends to New Year's Eve dinner to share the magnum with us.

Shortly before midnight, we eyed the last of the '55 still in the bottle. We grabbed it and antique flutes, and headed down the street, to the Pont des Arts, the very romantic bridge, which at that moment was totally packed with people of all ages and nationalities gathered to watch the Eiffel Tower light display. But as we sipped the last drops of the golden nectar the setting could not have felt more *intime:* it was us, the 1955, and the new millennium. The last taste was even more memorable than the first.

In America and many other nations wine is being consumed as never before. It has proved to be the element of French lifestyle that non-French peoples are most ready and willing to adopt. We have all heard about the healthful and rejuvenating effects of wine in moderation. In fact, wine is mankind's oldest medicine, first prescribed by Hippocrates in the fifth century B.C. Long before anyone had the slightest inkling that wine lowers bad cholesterol and elevates the good—before, in fact, cholesterol or anything less obvious than bile was known to affect our equilibrium—wine had recognized health benefits. It was killing pathogens and cleaning wounds before there was any awareness of bacteria. Or viruses: Did you care to know that the tannins in wine help prevent herpes and can speed the healing of fever sores? (Maybe not your problem, but still.) And it's always been known that wine aids digestion.

You can't go anywhere, it seems, without encountering some awareness of the "French Paradox": the French eat fatty foods such as *foie gras* and buttery croissants but have a lower rate of heart disease and live longer than most people in developed countries. The so-called paradox is easily explained by the habit of consuming wine in moderation along with those not-so-heart-healthy fats. The damage of "bad" fat is offset by the anticoagulants and antioxidants in wine. Wine keeps the circulatory system in good repair, and thus keeps the whole body younger. No one disagrees these days, but as recently as the 1970s, experts were burying the salubrious effects of wine. Partly this was due to a lack of understanding of how wine is a benefit. Partly, too, though, it was the legacy of temperance. In many cultures wine was better known not as good health in a glass, but as a debilitating intoxicant, which, despite its pleasures, would destroy the drinker who, meanwhile, would disturb the peace.

Research demonstrates that women who prefer wine (in moderation, of course) to beer, spirits, or abstinence live a healthier lifestyle and follow better dietary patterns than either abstainers or consumers of alcohol in other forms. Moderate wine drinkers live longer than abstainers, are better educated, and enjoy psychological benefits as well. It makes sense: wine is pleasurable and can help people relax and be in a good mood. Plus, it is generally consumed on social occasions, and sociability along with sound eating and drinking patterns is a proven boost to well-being.

Wine with its many ingredients, including important minerals, can be a tonic in several ways—there is even a clear though perhaps not causal relationship between drinking wine and high income. In America and France there is a common expression: "An apple a day keeps the doctor away." In Russia, however, they say: "Drink a glass of wine after your soup and you steal a ruble from your doctor."

THE PRESCRIPTION: *MODE D'EMPLOI*

Unlike other, newer medicines, wine doesn't come with a little crimped paper listing its active ingredients, cautioning about interactions and side effects, or recommending dosage. The prescription is simple. I like the Russian proverb because it sets wine in the context of the table, where it properly belongs. Wine is meant to be drunk always, always, always with food.

My French friends visiting New York are still shocked to see women gathered in a hotel lounge or a bar, drinking two or three glasses of Chardonnay on an empty stomach. Wine, being less alcoholic, may not hit you like hard liquor, but it will still go to your head after wreaking havoc on your unprotected stomach with a splash of acid.

I really don't drink except at mealtime, but if you must have a glass before dinner, be sure to have something to nibble with it. It won't throw off your caloric moderation if you choose the right foods and have just a little something. Proteins and fats are best. They slow the absorption process—not only of alcohol but of other foods, preventing overeating as well as tipsiness. For this reason any meal is well started with some slivers of cheese, salami, or some olives, of which you don't need more than four or five. Even a few nuts will do to protect your stomach. And as when one is trying to lose weight, preempt dehydration by drinking a glass or two of water half an hour before going out (alcohol is more than mildly dehydrating and diuretic).

BEGINNINGS

Brought up as a typical French girl of my generation, I started learning about wine at an early age. A family friend taught me at age six how to handle a Champagne flute (by the stem or foot) and on Sundays all the kids got a bit of wine mixed with water, as the ancients enjoyed theirs. By another mixed blessing, I was also introduced to Burgundy relatively early: in those days, the great *grands crus* and *premiers crus* Bourgogne did not cost that much. Now, however, indulging that pleasure can mean quite a hit in the *portefeuille*. I learned to locate on the map (and would later visit) all the little villages whose names were legend. My father had instilled in me a love of geography, though funnily enough, his own love was satisfied by books and maps, and he never left France except for one daytrip to England that itself became a family legend.

At special meals to celebrate a wedding, a birthday, or just the long Sunday lunch, I would linger around or under the table after dessert listening to heated conversations—or shall I say debates, French men being French men. That's when words such as *silky, velvety,* and *voluptuous* first entered my consciousness, together with the mysteries of the glassware. My parents' dear friend M. Lion, the big lion of a man who first taught me to hold the delicate Champagne glass, warned that any other vessel would break the spell of the magical wine, as in a fairy tale. On one occasion I remember a relative who had graduated from the École Polytechnique explaining rather technically just how the brain reconstructs the bouquet of a wine (or any food for that matter): integrating its look, feel, the context of the tasting, time of the day, and even one's mood. Our memory and many other psychological factors influence the way we judge a wine. Thus, the same wine never tastes the same twice. And compare notes as we might, we never really know how exactly the wine we are sipping tastes to someone else. Nevertheless, I do find that, as a rule, the better the company the better the wine tastes. French women don't drink alone.

And as the poet Paul Claudel observes, *"Le vin est le professeur du goût, le libérateur de l'esprit et l'illuminateur de l'intelligence"* (Wine teaches taste, frees the spirit, and illuminates one's intelligence).

You can't really learn wine from a book: all lessons are in the glass. You learn by tasting. You learn not only what you like but why you like it. Once that's established, you know when to drink it and with what. And along the way you learn about buying and storing, types and styles, glassware and accessories, and, of course, tasting. Plus there's pleasure in the glass. Pull some corks, pour some glasses, and continue your education. There are some things it helps to know before you remove the cork, however.

The Buy

Before approaching the sometimes bewildering business of choice, let's consider where to buy, and the basic caveat emptor.

Where do I go? Buy from a reputable seller who turns over stock regularly. There are great deals to be had at some large retailers that purchase in huge quantities at top discount or buy closeouts from wineries or distributors trying to raise cash or free up space for new inventory. These outlets are convenient and favor the consumer who knows what she or he wants and is content with some of the more popular brands. For more thoughtful selections, personal attention, and rare bottlings, wineshops and specialty retailers are recommended. And you can find good buys there as well. A knowledgeable shopkeeper will steer you to good vintages, which vary widely by geography (a bad year in the Rhône can be a fine year in Chile) and certainly by year (that year's Bordeaux may be the vintage of the century, while the next year's could be hard to give away—well, relatively hard). Someone who buys professionally can also sometimes point you to good wines in lesser vintages—the star of an otherwise lackluster year in Napa, say.

If you happen on a wine "promotion" featuring an improbably good price or a questionably exultant rave by the seller, there's a simple test. Buy a bottle. It's not a tech stock; the downside risk is small. If you like it, go back for another . . . even a case. Voilà: now you are a connoisseur and a collector. Most reputable stores won't steer you far wrong. You know where they live, and they want you back. Of course, taste is always subjective. But once you know each other's palate, any motivated seller and buyer can work together. Plus you'll find that people who work in these stores like wine and like talking about it—with you or anyone. (I know a bunch of guys who drop in each Saturday on their favorite wine store just to browse and chat.)

Buying direct from wineries, either on-site or via the Internet, is always good for a few bons mots at dinner: "When we were in Napa, we stopped by the So-and-So Estate and tried this heavenly Merlot. Well, we just had to bring back a few bottles." For many, such chitchat is part of the wine game. Sometimes the stories are quite entertaining, though the teller should always track the listener's attention and tolerance. There are other ways to socialize over a glass that are less self-reflexive. Wine always seems to lubricate the tongue.

How much should I spend? My second piece of advice about buying is no more "out there" than the first, but so many people can't seem to get it: price is not synonymous with quality. Truly great is one thing, greatly hyped quite another. There's no reason to get soaked. In today's global economy, with wine from dozens of regions around the world in distribution and new ones coming online each year, and modern production techniques yielding some amazing results, we are actually living through a time of wine glut, as near a buyer's market as I've seen. For the price of this book, you can easily find a terrific bottle of wine. The "sweet spot" of value I look for nowadays is the quality bottle between $9 and $29 retail. No doubt there are decent ones to be had for less, but the odds of finding them are against you, and the cheap disappointments can add up as you taste your way to a winner. I certainly buy and drink wines well above $30 (professional development, right?). Are they "worth it"? Quite often they are, and I have spent years building an experienced palate capable of appreciating subtle traits. But I also know what I'm paying for: the supply-and-demand effect that kicks in when a large segment of the market wants the same product; the middleman who buys and stores the wine until it's old enough to command top dollar and reaching its peak. Of course, top expertise and unique wines also command a premium and do often yield greatness, but after a certain point other factors contribute to cost above any standard of quality.

In the course of my career, I have been the president of one ultrapremium winery in California and chaired the board of another. Both estates produce exceptional wines (if I do say so myself), for a price still within my sweet spot, though at the upper end. But minding the books, I knew that the costs of a bottle were largely buried in the vineyards. Suitable real estate in wine country can make Manhattan prices seem reasonable, as I discovered firsthand when we decided to expand into new acreage and plant more vines. So we borrowed the money.

And guess who is paying the interest and principal on the loan, bottle by bottle?

At least in California there is *some* room to grow. Consider two of my favorite wines, Champagne and red Burgundy. Both are dependent on harvests of Pinot Noir vineyards, some of them postage-stamp small. As there is no immediate prospect of change in the consensus that wines from these regions are among the world's best, the grapes lovingly coaxed to fullness on these little tracts of land are likely to remain the most expensive fruits on earth.

Okay, so what should I get? There are so many choices. Overall, that's a good thing. Huge choice, however, has its downside, too. But learning with wine is trial and error. Again, don't sweat it: you are not picking mutual funds. We begin with the simplest facts: Wines are either sparkling or still. They are white, rosé, or red. They are dry, slightly sweet, or sweet. They are all made from grapes. Here's where it gets a little complicated.

There are dozens and dozens of grape varieties from which wine is made. And those grapes don't even taste quite the same when grown in two different areas of the same vineyard, let alone in two different parts of the world. Furthermore, while great wine is made in the vineyards, there are techniques employed in the winery that can make a huge difference to what ends up in your glass. Some techniques are officially prescribed (those controlled appellations, again): a wine labeled from this region will be not less than x percent Cabernet Sauvignon, not more than y percent Merlot, for instance. Yes, as if the dozens of grapes were not mind-boggling enough, the game is further complicated by the fact that some wines are blends (named for place, such as Bordeaux), while others are varietals, named for the grape of which they are mainly constituted, such as Merlot.

Like most people, I'm far more interested in flavor than in production specs, so when choosing, I work backward from taste, which is also how I advise you to get started if you are a relative novice. Start by buying varietals (one-grape) wines within the price sweet spot.

Get to know the grapes, and you are on your way. Where to start? Let's go to the head of the class: the so-called vinifera, those grapes that dominate and compete head-on for market share in the global wine business.

White grapes: the Chardonnay and the Sauvignon Blanc rule, but don't neglect to try a Pinot Grigio from Italy or a Pinot Gris from Oregon or a Riesling from Alsace.

The reds: Cabernet Sauvignon, Merlot, Pinot Noir, and Syrah make up the lion's share (but that list excludes four grapes found in some of my favorite wines: Zinfandel from California, Grenache from the southern Rhône, Nebbiolo from Piedmont, and Sangiovese from Tuscany).

Once you know a Cabernet from a Pinot Noir, a Chardonnay from a Sauvignon Blanc, you can go on to explore the wines in which different grapes are blended, wines more often named not for grapes but for regions, such as a familiar little blend called Champagne. As I have mentioned, it depends on the Pinot Noir, which is a red grape. You might be scratching your head: Isn't Champagne a white wine? Another French Paradox? Not so much: Champagne typically contains the juice of both red and white grapes, mostly Pinot Noir and Chardonnay. But grape juice is clear; it's the grape skin that furnishes color, and only if it's left in contact with the juice (not the case with Champagne).

Incidentally, when you are exploring wines, it helps to keep a journal, recording your impressions of things you've tried. Many wine lovers soak off the labels and paste them in a diary. (Looking back on wine adventures past, one never wonders where all the years went.)

Here's another eye-opener: A wine that is arguably the world's best (and certainly one of the most expensive) is made from a grape I haven't even mentioned—the Sémillon. I am referring to the greatest of all dessert wines, Château d'Yquem [dee-KEM]. Some upscale restaurants offer it on occasion by the glass, making tasting it almost affordable—well, an affordable luxury anyway. If you ever have the good fortune to taste this divine elixir, the last thing on your mind will be what grape it's made from. It's all in the glass, and the more you know . . . well, you know.

A final word about choosing: Palates new to wine often prefer semisweet, if not sweet, though they soon acquire a taste for dry wines. Likewise, though white is more often the starting point than red, white wine drinkers often end up as red aficionadas.

Storage

Wine is meant for drinking, not storing. In France, just as in America and the rest of the world, most wines are consumed within hours of their purchase. Restaurants have to plan ahead, so if you order a bottle of wine and find it costs twice as much as what you've paid for it retail, be advised that not all the restaurateur's markup is profit: you are paying for the bottle's acquisition as well as for proper storage to ensure that it hasn't become "cooked" and maderized (spoiled by heat) and is served at the proper temperature. Even so, most restaurants don't carry a large (and costly) inventory of wines but replenish most of their stock weekly or monthly from a distributor.

Operating on a need-to-drink basis, the average consumer buys a bottle (or two if she's having company). Many buy a bottle to bring when invited for dinner (sometimes a better choice of house gift than flowers, which inevitably send the hosts scrambling in search of an empty vase). Discovering a wine you like, you may buy several bottles. But in most cases, you still don't have a storage issue. Most wines for sale are the current release and vintage, meant not to be laid down and aged but to be consumed. Proper conditions for short-term storage are easy: if the room or space is not too hot or cold for human comfort (say, between 50 and 90 degrees), the wine will be comfortable, too.

If wines are to be kept for months or even years—you may like to have the same one again on your next anniversary, say—above all keep them in a dark place (light is one of wine's enemies) and protected from sudden, dramatic temperature fluctuations. (The 50- to 90-degree interval is still okay, provided the wine doesn't suffer an unseasonable swing from low to high in a matter of hours.) When in doubt, err on the cold side. Consistent cold down to near freezing is not a problem, but high heat can be fatal.

If you are storing a few bottles or more in a closet or cabinet, store horizontally to keep the cork moist and prevent it from shrinking and oxidizing the wine prematurely. You don't need a wine rack, though it can be helpful when trying to remove one bottle without agitating the others at rest. If you find you are regularly holding twenty-five bottles or more, you might invest in a wine refrigerator, or *cave*. The smallest countertop models can be had for around $200. Under-the-counter units are pricier and take up the space of a dishwasher. If you find yourself holding 250 bottles, you will probably know this already: you should definitely consider investing in a *cave*. Some of them are as large as an armoire and cost several thousand dollars. It's not cheap, but weigh the cost relative to your investment in the wine: 250 bottles can represent quite an outlay. And with variable climate zones that can be set to suit the ideal storage temperature of any type of wine, these units can provide some peace of mind to the more ambitious collector. We use them, and they keep the whites ready to drink and the reds at a temperature to ensure graceful aging.

The Pour

For me, there's little doubt that some wine-tasting rituals and props enhance the experience, as proper napkins and changing plates for each course can do at the dinner table. Glassware is not a luxury, it's essential. A good all-purpose eight-ounce glass will do, although you should never pour more than four to six ounces into it. Such a "sommelier's glass" is fine for whites, reds, and even sparkling wines. It should be tapered at the top to capture the aromas but without too long a stem, which can cause instability. Molded glass will do, though crystal can enhance the discernment and appreciation of color and has a delicate feel on the lips that can also enhance pleasure.

The glass makers and wine magazines tout the benefits of glasses designed for each specific wine type. It's not nonsense:

a larger balloon bowl, for instance, does help capture the more abundant bouquets, and there are shapes designed to make the wine flow into your mouth in some optimal way. Most of these refinements have little bearing on the basic enjoyment of wine, though. Yes, a red Burgundy, with its complex aromas, benefits from the big balloon. Yes, the tulip shape of a Champagne flute keeps the bubbles bubbling longer and the bursting bouquet concentrated (so you should *immediately* junk those saucer-shaped Champagne glasses apocryphally said to be modeled on the shape of Marie Antoinette's breasts!). And generally a heavy glass with a long stem feels precarious in my hand. Lately, stemless glasses with bowls of various sizes (larger for reds, smaller for whites) have come into fashion. I rather like them. A nice modern, casually elegant touch, they are our glass of choice in the country.

A word about washing: Glassware should of course be clean, but use only the very minimum of detergent, rinse very well, and air dry—don't use a dishcloth reeking of fabric softener. Many a wine experience is doomed by odors already in the glass.

A corkscrew is the one other essential for wine after a glass, though it may not be for much longer. Corks are traditional, of course, but are in short supply and often are flawed or "bad"—up to one in twenty bottles at times—and impart off flavors, sometimes to the point of making the wine unpleasant and unacceptable. Synthetic corks are making good inroads and are effective. Moreover, with so much wine consumed within a year of bottling, screw tops are finding a place, especially among white wines, in the low and middle quality ranges. Fine by me.

The cork and corkscrew, though, are part of the ritual of wine and are standard for fine wines, as they have been for centuries. There's even a rich tradition of collecting corkscrews, notably old silver contraptions that penetrated many a venerable neck (and cork). Modern technology has improved the corkscrew and made the job easier. I advise investing in a good one that should last you for life, even if it doesn't become a collectible or heirloom. What's a good corkscrew? One you find easy to use. It's all about the screw, which is called the worm. It should look like a coil and not a screw, and nowadays the most efficient are coated with Teflon. The best-known brand is Screwpull, but there are worthy competitors. We generally use one of the lever types, partly because we tend to open bottles regularly, but any model with a good worm works well and easily. There's a certain machismo about the purity of the basic waiter's corkscrew—fine if you can handle one with ease—but such considerations don't concern French women.

To Decant or Not to Decant

Before removing the cork, you must make sure you have the serving temperature right. It's not necessarily the same as the storage temperature. And if you are following the 50 Percent Solution and refrigerating half a bottle (see page 25), you can't just plop it straight onto the table like a two-liter bottle of Coke (which, anyway, I hope you are not still drinking). The rules are pretty simple: Champagne and white wines should be chilled to between 45 and 55 degrees. Overchilled wine will not release its aromas, so chill minimally. The rule of thumb with red wines is room temperature (take the half bottle out of the refrigerator half an hour or so before serving), but this centuries-old rule predates central heating and assumes a room temperature of 65 degrees (a good pouring temperature for reds). If your room is 80 or 90 degrees, serve the wine at the temperature of the cool, dark place where you've been keeping it—somewhere in the 60s is a good target.

Decanting is another ritual about which there are strong opinions. There really are only two reasons to decant: sedimentation and aeration. But my practice runs against orthodoxy in respect to both: I mostly decant younger wines and serve older wines from their bottle.

Decanters are lovely things, of course. They shine and glitter and look good on shelves. But an old wine bottle or a $5 glass decanter or pitcher is all you need.

You may have observed a sommelier carefully pouring wine from a bottle while illuminating the neck with a candle (rare nowadays). So mystical, when a little flashlight would work fine—the point being to make sure sediments remain in the bottle and don't make their way into the decanter and your glass and ultimately your mouth. Sedimentary deposition occurs not only in riverbeds; it occurs naturally in big reds as they age and their tannins (the naturally occurring chemicals that account for the astringency of wine) soften. Nothing bad will happen to you if you ingest the sediment, but it can interfere with the pleasure of drinking.

The second reason for decanting is to "awaken" a sleeping wine through aeration. Wine is a living, breathing thing during its time in the bottle and in the glass. It is always changing, especially in the glass. A little oxygen can really open up and release the flavors in a complex wine, as well as mellow the rougher edges of immaturity (again the tannins, necessary for structure but also responsible for harshness: wine can't live with 'em, can't live without 'em).

The problem with decanting very old wines is that they often die in the decanter, oxidizing too quickly, before you can enjoy them. That's why we prefer to stand the bottle up for a day, letting the sediment fall to the bottom; then, after opening, we take care not to pour the dregs into the glass (think of it as decanting straight into the glass). But who has lots of old bottles of wine to decant anyway? It's the big, youngish red wines that most of us uncork and find too rowdy to drink without a few breaths or hours of air. When we were newer to wine, we played the game of tracking the taste of a wine from its first awakening when uncorked through its maturity and finally death, when the air has robbed it of all its most pleasing characteristics. In some sense a wine becomes a different wine at each stage of this life of hours. Talk about the fullness of time.

The Taste

Now we're talking. Here's where it all comes together. All the knowledge about grapes and paraphernalia is but an adjunct to the ultimate business of tasting. In tasting you discover your, well, taste: your personal style and preferences in relation to wine. But this shouldn't be a static pleasure. I know a woman who orders a Sancerre regardless of what she's eating, rain or shine. After the film *Sideways* was released, Pinot Noir became the default wine of many people who had sipped Merlot for years. Never drink wine by default. Knowing what you like is one thing, being closed to new experiences quite another.

As with any aesthetic experience, it does help to be informed and thoughtful about what you are looking for, so you can say not just I like this, but I like this *because.* In that causal link is the difference between the child's and the adult's taste. In helping you become usefully systematic about your wine appreciation, let's *faire simple.* As I and so many others do, you can look for the four classic characteristics: color, aroma (aka nose), taste, and finish. Each tells you something and is a subsidiary pleasure in the enjoyment of the whole. Nothing teaches you to coordinate the use of your senses like wine tasting. And as the senses are the gateways to pleasure, consider the tasting of wine your total-fitness sensory work-out. If you can do it well with wine, you can do it with anything and reap the benefits of sensation rather than quantity. Real wine lovers don't get fat.

Before tasting a wine, examine its *color* (the appearance and color is called *la robe*—the dress). Pour a small amount into a clear glass. No matter the color of the wine, it must be clear, even brilliant, certainly not cloudy or with suspended particles. The clarity of color is a tip-off to quality, a well-made wine, but also to the type of grape and the age of the wine. You can tell a Pinot Noir, for example, from a Cabernet Sauvignon because it is generally lighter in color. Its grape skins have less pigment than some of the bigger reds, which can be almost purple when young. If you tilt the glass slightly and set it against a white background, you can get a good sense of the true color and hue by looking from the deeper center out to the thinnest edge where the wine laps the glass.

Brilliance, especially in white wines, indicates acidity, without which a wine gets "flabby" (yes, even wine is not immune). Also in white wines, colorlessness indicates immaturity; pale yellow with green overtones suggests a very young to young wine with a good acidity. When a wine is of age, one can expect hues of straw to gold-yellow. Copper-gold also means a mature wine; amber may indicate oxidation, and wine that could well be past its prime.

Among reds, the young'uns are marked by their violet-purple hue; cherry red suggests a wine grown-up enough to drink but one you could keep a while longer; red-orange means the wine is maturing or mature and surely drinking near its peak. Reddish-brown suggests an aged wine fast getting past it, so *carpe vinum*. Brown means a very old wine, which may still please, but it's not a good bet. We've had some very old Bordeaux that had lost perhaps two thirds of their color, and the remaining hue was brown indeed, but some of those wines were still showing fruit (the remnants of youth that in good wine are metamorphosed by age into the complexities of bouquet). They were oozing pleasure, not least that of drinking history.

Once you master these color codes, you'll find they are not nearly as anxious-making as Homeland Security's. And it's amazing how much you can learn by sight alone.

Another visual element can tell you the amount of alcohol in the wine: we call this looking at its legs. To do this, you swirl the wine in the glass a couple of times (hold the stem between thumb and index finger, and make some little circles on or near the tabletop). Where the lapping wine has coated the inside of the glass it "tears" back down into the bowl. The speed and thickness of those legs indicate viscosity, which means more alcohol. A high-proof Amarone, for instance, will have much more serious legs (thicker, slower) than, say, most Merlot.

Swirling is also the segue to smelling the wine. And aroma more than anything reveals flavor. Tasting is mainly confirmation. (Going to a wine tasting with a head cold is therefore like going to the shoe department without your credit card: you'll never get what you came for.) A little swirl releases the wine's aroma, which you should quickly draw into your nose, either in a long, slow draught or in a few (inaudible) sniffs—don't vacuum the glass, just get enough to bring the aroma in contact with your olfactory organ. First impressions are especially revealing when "nosing" a wine, as when tasting it. With practice you will be able to tell several things from the wine's nose, including its age, complexity, fruit, flavor characteristics, and overall quality. But first and foremost: if the nose gives you pleasure, chances are you will enjoy drinking the wine.

Actually *tasting* wine has its little techniques as well. The key is to take a sip and let it roll throughout your mouth and over your tongue, alighting on as many of your flavor receptors (taste buds) as possible. Do it right and it's like 3-D imaging. Serious tasters do two more things. With the wine in their mouths, they pull in some air through their lips and over the wine to increase vaporization and aeration. Then they sort of chew the wine in an attempt to get at any flavors that might be too subtle or incipient.

Finally, you pick up more flavors through your mouth and nose as you swallow and again when you exhale. This is to examine the all-important *finish,* and what you look for is *length,* duration of sensation: the more complex the lingering flavors, the longer they persist. Wines with a so-called short finish, such as simple whites, can give pleasure, but for the orgasmic wine enthusiast the real mind-blowing pleasure is in the overtones and complexities, the apprehension of structure, and the experience of length.

At that point, you've tasted the wine and are ready for drinking, so *Santé,* as the French say: to your health!

As I've said, describing experience is one way of augmenting it. It's true you can't *describe* the effect of a sunset upon the senses, or of a wine for that matter. But you can describe the various attributes that contribute to the sensation of what you are drinking. Much pretentious vocabulary arises here. I avoid it. Only you and perhaps those with whom you enjoy wine need share a lingua franca. The point is not pretension but to encourage mindfulness by making the experience more conscious, less passive, and thereby more intense. The best things in life can pass you by if you aren't paying attention. It's easier to hold on to a memory if you can remember its parts: if you know the trees by name, you can recall not just a pretty vista but a particular landscape. A great wine will not hit you over the head with its greatness; you have to explore and map it, seek it out where it lurks.

WHEN IN SONOMA, DO AS THE SONOMANS DO

Before agritourism became an "in" thing, Edward and I systematically traveled to many of the world's famous vineyards, continuing the geography game I had begun to play as a girl. The point was not just pilgrimage for its own sake; we wanted to drink the local wines with the local food. It's no coincidence that the two typically work wonderfully well together. Often the locals have been working on these marriages for centuries. And tasting and dining at the source is a great way to learn not only about wine and food, but also about history and the cultural context that gave rise to the local gastronomic style.

Drinking local is something I recommend highly. If in Sonoma, drink Sonoma; if in Burgundy, drink Burgundy. It's part of the unique pleasure of slipping entirely into the local lifestyle. In this way, we live seasonally even though wine is not really seasonal: summer in Provence is not a time to drink great Bordeaux. There are plenty of choices from among the dozen good wineries surrounding our village and hundreds in the region. Of course we do have our preferences, and uncannily the wines we prefer are always made by the winemakers we like best.

One Provençal specialty I appreciate when in Provence (though rarely in New York or Paris) is still rosé, always served chilled in France whenever the sun is shining and the sea is visible. In the South of France—in Provence or on the Riviera—rosés are the apéritif of choice. Not surprisingly, they are produced in these areas and throughout the southern Rhône Valley. And they go exceptionally well with the olives and other munchies the locals traditionally enjoy before a meal. It's a ritual you'll see at all the starred restaurants in Provence but almost nowhere in the middle and north of France.

As with all rules, however, the drink-local principle has its exceptions. We were at a restaurant in Alsace with an incredible selection of local wines, which, though mainly limited to white, do go remarkably well with Alsatian food (and, yes, we did start with a dry Riesling). But looking through the wine list, we noticed a few choice bottles from Bordeaux and Burgundy, some startlingly great vintages and labels—and at prices as close to bargains as such wines come. It was some years ago, but the memory is strong: we picked a '76 DRC Grands Echézeaux. Because most visitors do observe the drink-local rule, wines from outside a region often don't sell and so remain on the wine list a long while, sometimes for years, without a price increase. This was one of those situations. The price was a blast from the past, although the wine was never drinking better.

When the staff of a good restaurant recognize that you have spotted a terrific value on their wine list, their eyes see differently. A kinship of pleasure is immediately established. We've observed that a good wine choice—even a bargain—can result in super-special treatment, often ending in the exchange of stories and a tasting of a "mystery" glass of wine with cheese or dessert. Ultimately, great restaurateurs are not in it for the money—or at least not *only* for the money.

The wine industry is a hospitality industry as well. We have met so many generous people, some of whom work miracles. I'll never forget our first visit to the Tuscan estate of Capezzana. The lovely vineyard and winery near Florence, with its Medici villa, is still one of the grand Old World emblems, where tradition, family, ritual, and seasonality effortlessly entwine into the fabric of life. Sublime art carries the experience well beyond the threshold of civility. The domain is splendid, nestled in the hills, the Duomo of Florence visible in the far distance. We were welcomed by one of the daughters, who served as the oenologist and pizza expert in the small cooking school the family also run. She was eager to show us the cellar, but her brother, the vineyard manager, appeared and wanted first to show us where it all began. No sooner had we set down our bags than we were staring at the majestic plain ringed by olive groves, the pigs in their pen, and stray chickens scratching here and there, as heedless of the history as of the beauty of the chapel where the eldest daughter (head of marketing) was married.

At dinner, the first half hour was spent on the terrace with the count and countess, a couple in their eighties whose stamina and joie de vivre would shame most of the young go-getters I know in New York. With great anticipation we headed across the courtyard to the dining room, where the chef, a local, had prepared simple but splendid antipasti and pastas, then meat, accompanied by wines of the property. The food, wine, and setting produced a set of sensations I will never replicate, no matter how many bottles of Capezzana I drink. This is because everything was of the place. On the estate was also a semi-subsistence farm that had produced almost everything we ate. Every member of the family had a job, whether in the fields, in the kitchen, in the smokehouse, or in the office, and each seemed enlivened by his labors. Such a place is a rarity, but rarer still, I reflected, is how the luxury of enjoying such elementally satisfying work—the toil of creating pleasures—is almost as rewarding as enjoying the fruits. The count, though past his toiling days, was a wonderful raconteur, and the countess looked to please in all sorts of subtle ways. The next morning after waking in a room decorated with Della Robbia ceramics, we were met at breakfast by a gorgeous lemon cake made with olive oil, fresh from the oven. I remembered that at dinner we had been discoursing on the pleasures of the French *tarte au citron,* in the course of which exchange the countess had evidently registered that lemon has a magical taste for me.

After a morning soaking in the daylight on the terrace,

peering at the Duomo in the distance, one further pleasure remained to us: a lunch of farm-fresh peas, fava beans mixed with prosciutto in a perfect pasta dish, and the culmination— a homemade biscotti and a sip of the estate's *vin santo,* the sweet "holy wine" made since medieval times. The grapes are traditionally pressed during the week before Easter after drying on straw since October. The divine nectar, produced in tiny quantities, matures up to ten years after fermentation and is offered to honored guests. A lot of effort and cost. Is it worth it? It is a miracle by any standard of wine.

Not every winery is a Medici estate and palazzo, and my visit to the celebrated Cloudy Bay in New Zealand bears witness to that fact. No aristocrats and no Della Robbias, but lots of sheep. Named after the nearby body of water, Cloudy Bay is in Marlborough, nestled amid a cluster of vineyards and open country, comfortable, unassuming homes, and relaxed, friendly people. Although many other wineries make beautiful wines, Cloudy Bay still is the point of reference and has even become the stuff of myth. We love the taste—not grassy or overly vegetal like some Sauvignon Blancs but full of exotic fruits, including lychee. This is a New World structure, a combination of power and personality. And there's almost a scrubbed cleanliness to this perfectly made wine. It tastes healthy. Plus it marries exceptionally with food, say grilled or sautéed fish with some fresh asparagus. The purity and flavor of the ingredients in the simple but elegantly cooked meals we experienced in and around Cloudy Bay, along with the friendliness of everyone we met, is what we drink every time we pull a cork of Cloudy Bay. What a bottle!

. . .

Most wine experiences, however, are not in Tuscan villas or on the other side of the world but at home or in restaurants, where variety is more important to encouraging conviviality than the quantity. I was reminded of this recently when out on a "girls' night" in New York, celebrating a birthday. We started with a glass of bubbly. For the main course two of us wanted a white wine and two a red, so I quickly realized that I had to help with the choices, as they were my guests and not as familiar with the bistro's well-chosen list. Of course, the sommelier is a great help for situations like this. But knowing the taste of the two friends who'd ordered the soft-shell crab, I recommended a white from the Loire for one and a Santenay, a red Burgundy that was both light and relatively inexpensive, for the other. A third friend, who loves Italian wine, picked a nice Chianti Classico Riserva from Monsanto that suited her lamb beautifully. As for the birthday girl, she chose to have her quail with more bubbly. I made the choice for some, others chose for themselves, but each tried a new wine and came away with a name to remember on her next visit to the wine store.

WHEN IN DOUBT, HAVE CHAMPAGNE

I am not alone in the belief that there's a fail-safe wine choice you could always make, depending, of course, on your budget. Champagne, an extremely versatile wine, came to be known as the "wine of kings" because, for centuries, the coronation of French kings took place in the great cathedral at Reims, the capital of Champagne, about ninety minutes northeast of Paris. Ever since, it has reigned as the wine not only of sovereignty but of love, romance, and celebration. Perhaps that status owes something to its natural traces of lithium. (No, it won't cure clinical depression, but it may well help one's mood: imbibers of bubbly get bubbly themselves, and just a glass will do the trick.) For me, Champagne is a state of mind.

For the record, Champagne should *not* give you a headache (though I suppose if you drink it by the quart anything's possible). It's actually the kindest of wines, lowest in histamines and calories while full of healthy minerals. So many people tell me they can't drink Champagne, but upon interrogation it comes out that they've been drinking something else. Champagne, the one and only, comes from the Champagne region of France. The usual culprit in these head cases is cheap, sweet sparkling wine from California, Italy, Spain, or even France, but not from Champagne. The low-cost bubbles sometimes get passed off as Champagne at big wedding-reception toasts. A glass or two of that decoction of sugar, mediocre grapes, and shoddy vinification would give anyone a headache. A polite sip for the toast is plenty.

By law, real Champagne is the most quality-controlled wine on earth. The white grape Chardonnay and the reds Pinot Noir and Pinot Meunier are gathered from different villages and even different years to be blended by the cellar master. When the wine in the bottle is from a single, exceptional year, though, that's a vintage Champagne, which is then aged from three to five years before being released. But 85 percent of all Champagne is nonvintage (or multivintage, if you will) and bears no year on the label; the cellar master is not dependent on any one harvest and so can maintain the wine's consistency and quality. Besides the vintage and nonvintage Champagne, a small percentage of a premium vintage goes into what is known as a *prestige cuvée,* such as Dom Pérignon or Veuve Clicquot's La Grande Dame. These are the best bottles the Champagne houses make.

Each house has its style, largely due to the grape composition of the house blend. Some are fuller-bodied, generally indicating a blend that is two-thirds red grapes. A small number of houses use only Chardonnay, and this is called Blanc de Blancs (white from white). Some Champagnes are rosés (that's a Clicquot specialty), which generally include a little red wine in the blend. Champagne's soul, however, is in its famous bubbles, which result from a second fermentation in the bottle. Just before the cork is inserted and the label affixed, the bottle is topped up with reserved wine and sugar; this allows the fermentation to continue and lets the cellar master adjust the sweetness of the wine. Brut is the driest, Extra Dry (despite its name) is a little sweeter, and Demi-sec (half dry) is sweet.

Oscar Wilde said that only those without imagination can't find a good reason to drink Champagne. French women can always think of something.

THE MARRIAGE OF WINE AND FOOD

This shouldn't be the last word in a chapter on wine: it should be the first, second, and third. Pursuers of the joie de vivre and the *art de vivre* know this. Wine's essential identity as food is fully realized only in the sacrament of its marriage with other foods. No true lover of wine would content herself with such pleasure as could be had by drinking alone, without food or company. She understands that in the calculus of pleasures, the whole exceeds the sum of its parts. It's a case of $1 + 1 = 11$, not 2. But such dividends can be earned only by active management of pleasure.

Some marriages of food and wine are classic and time-tested, others are idiosyncratic, but either way you will know a great experience when you have one. For a classic, try a Sauternes with a blue cheese, preferably Roquefort. The blessings of culture: you could have drunk for a lifetime without discovering that one on your own. As an example of the idiosyncratic, one of my personal favorite discoveries is Champagne and pizza. All types of pizza. I love it. In the spirit of improbable unions that somehow work wonderfully, let's consider the two most basic rules of food-and-wine pairing. Rule One: Drink red wine with meat and white wine with fish and poultry. Rule Two: Forget Rule One. Gastronomic norms are helpful, but they are only derivations of experience, not prescriptions. Nothing can trump the "wow" moment you experience for yourself.

Of course, wine is a limited resource and not cheap. It is indeed possible to choose wrong, or at least to make one choice far worse than another. The French don't believe that all pairings are valid any more than they believe all children are bright. Quality is about degrees of difference. So what follows is not a set of prescriptions but, I hope, a framework allowing you to operate according to individual taste while avoiding common pitfalls. Life's too short for a Shiraz-and-poached-Dover-sole experiment (though it beats any Coca-Cola pairing). For professionals, food-and-wine pairings can get insanely complicated—accounting for grape, region, vintage, and style in relation to each single food item. Then a change of sauce and all bets are off. As in all things, I seek pleasure in simplicity.

The simplest plan is to drink one wine throughout the meal. Select one that goes best with the main course and is at least not wildly at odds with any of the others. (At a restaurant, I recommend you choose your main course, *then* settle on the wine, then decide on your starter—that is, pair the wine to food and then pair the remaining food selections to the wine.) As I write this, I am in Beverly Hills, and last evening I dined at Spago and drank a full-bodied Champagne throughout the meal; it was superb with the duck main course and a fine complement to the fish appetizer. For multiwine, multicourse dinners, a good rule of thumb is to proceed from light to full-bodied wines, and/or from young to old. So that perhaps means a white wine, then a red (white after red is actually extremely rare and usually comes up because of a cheese or dessert choice). So you might see: Champagne (peerless apéritif), white wine, red wine. Or perhaps, under even fancier circumstances, Champagne, white wine, young red wine, old red wine, dessert wine.

The notion of holding back the older wines upends a rule at least as old as the New Testament. At the marriage at Cana, the best wines were expected to be served first, before the guests got sloshed and could not appreciate them. And so there was general surprise when the wine Jesus made from water was served late in the meal and proved to be better than the wine served earlier. Nowadays we know that pleasures should build as a meal progresses—no anticlimaxes. And drinking too much too soon negates pleasure, though don't hold back your best wine or wine-and-food pairing till your palate is fatigued.

White or sparkling wine is usually best with starters. With *antipasto* perhaps a Pinot Grigio, Pinot Gris, or Sauvignon Blanc. With *sushi or tuna carpaccio,* Champagne or Sauvignon Blanc. *Asparagus and artichokes* have a pronounced effect on wine, making it taste sweeter, and so are tricky to pair: try a grassy Sauvignon Blanc with citric overtones, and don't pull out your best bottle with either of these. With *caviar?* Champagne, *bien sûr. Oysters?* Chablis, Muscadet, Champagne, or sparkling wine; depending on the type and style of oyster, perhaps a Pinot Gris or Sauvignon Blanc. Ditto for *clams* (raw or casino). With *crudités,* something like Pinot Blanc, Chenin Blanc, or a light Chardonnay. With *foie gras,* Champagne or sparkling wine, or a late-harvest Riesling or Sauternes. *Nuts or olives?* Champagne or another dry sparkling wine. *Prosciutto and melon* offer interesting possibilities, starting with my favorite, Muscat Beaumes-de-Venise. A Pinot Blanc can go well. *Quiche?* Chardonnay, Viognier, Riesling, or sparkling wine. *Scallops* call for Sauvignon Blanc, Chardonnay, sparkling wines, or Sémillon. *Smoked fish* (trout, herring), on the other hand, can marry well with Riesling, Gewürztraminer, Pinot Blanc, and sparkling wine.

Soups call for no wine at all. *Salads* are difficult for wine because of the dressings, especially those that are vinegar-based. Your best bet apart from water is a Sauvignon Blanc, especially if it is a full salad, like a Niçoise.

Say *"pasta,"* even in a salad, and I think light Chianti. A pasta salad can also work with a Sémillon or a light red. *Pâtés* marry with a range of wines from Gewürztraminer to sparkling wines to Pinot Gris to Beaujolais. For pasta as an appetizer or main course, it depends on the sauce and ingredients. If it's a shellfish pasta, a white, for sure, say Pinot Grigio, Pinot Gris, Vernaccio di San Gimignano, Chardonnay, Sauvignon Blanc, or Pinot Blanc. For a pasta with vegetables, a Sauvignon Blanc, Pinot Blanc, Pinot Grigio, Pinot Gris, Vernaccio di San Gimignano, or a Barbera work for me. A cream sauce calls for the acidity of a Chardonnay or Pinot Blanc, among a range of whites. And, *finalemente,* pasta with tomato sauce. Did you say Chianti? Perhaps a Rosso di Montepulciano, Zinfandel, or Côtes du Rhône. (Avoid anything old, because tomato sauces interact too much with wine to permit subtle flavors to survive.)

Red wines are the choice with *cured cold meats,* such as salami, prosciutto, chorizo, and Serrano ham. Ditto beef carpaccio. Try Chianti, Barbera, or, for a bigger red, a Ribera del Duero. (Bigness is full body, depth of flavor, and sometimes overpowering for the less experienced palate.) *Lighter cold meats,* such as chicken, marry well with a Pinot Gris, Riesling, Beaujolais, or other light red.

Fish and Shellfish

Lobster cries out to me for Chardonnay from Burgundy or the Napa Valley. I can also enjoy it with a top Chablis—or Champagne: I couldn't count the number of lobsters we've boiled on a Sunday evening in New York and washed down with bubbly. *Crab* can match with a Sauvignon Blanc as well as Chardonnay and Champagne. *Mussels,* among my favorites, go down nicely with a Muscadet, Pinot Gris, Pinot Blanc, Chenin Blanc, or perhaps a Spanish Albariño. A light and simple Chardonnay, like a Saint-Véran, can work, too, but as with most seafood, a white with a little acidity (or "backbone") meets the challenge for me. With *shrimp* try a Riesling, Pinot Grigio, Pinot Gris, Pinot Blanc, or Sauvignon Blanc. For fish of delicate taste such as *red snapper or striped bass,* Chardonnay is more the rule than exception: I'm there nine out of ten times, though, depending on the sauce and accompaniments, a Riesling, Pinot Blanc, or Viognier can work too, as with other white fish. We are red wine partisans, particularly of Pinot Noir, when it comes to everybody's heart-healthy favorite, *salmon.* Red's my choice for *tuna* as well, perhaps a Merlot, though you could also consider a Sauvignon Blanc, Pinot Gris, or Chardonnay, in that order. *Swordfish* works for me with the same lineup, though I can also enjoy it with sparkling wine, especially rosé Champagne. As for *sushi,* which I adore, a white such as a Riesling, Sancerre, or Sauvignon Blanc will be fine, but for me nothing beats sparkling wine.

Meat and Poultry

Chicken has the reputation of going well with almost any wine, white or red, but here I have a strong preference for a red from the southern Rhône. Rotisserie chicken is one of Edward's favorite dishes, so we have it regularly in Paris, in Provence, and also at home in New York. We always have it with a Côtes du Rhône, a Gigondas, or on occasion a Châteauneuf du Pape. Having spent my adult life coming to these preferences, I can't think of a reason to change. Now, if we are sitting in some star-laden gastronomic temple and are served chicken in a preparation that disguises its identity as such, we would probably set aside our homely preferences and opt for an elegant Chardonnay or more likely a white Châteauneuf du Pape.

Any of these whites or a Pinot Noir would be my pick for

Cornish hen. Duck means red, Pinot Noir being my first choice. Memories of the duck at Paris's La Tour d'Argent with great bottles of Burgundy have pretty much set my standard. Still, lots of people enjoy a Merlot or Cabernet Sauvignon with their duck; and truth be told, the occasional Saint-Émilion (a Bordeaux combining both those grapes plus Cabernet Franc) has indeed passed my lips at a duck dinner. Ditto Barbaresco. *Pheasant* means Pinot Noir or perhaps a Syrah. And I think I am on to something with rosé Champagne. *Quail* calls for only Pinot Noir. *Goose* can get it on with some bigger red wines, spicy Rhônes first of all. Then there is *turkey:* every Thanksgiving you read wine suggestion after suggestion. For Thanksgiving roast turkey, a patriotic California Zinfandel is our pick by a country mile. A Barbaresco is tempting, however, as is a Pinot Noir. A really big white Chardonnay can work, but we prefer that only with straight white-meat turkey, especially in a sandwich.

Veal, like chicken, is wine flexible, and Chardonnay is recommended, though a light red is understandable. *Pork* with fuller flavor can sometimes work with a big white, like a white Châteauneuf du Pape, but my preference is for a medium-bodied red, such as a Merlot or Spanish Tempranillo. A *light-meat pork dish* can go with a fruity white, such as a German Riesling or a Viognier. Plain *rabbit* calls first for a white, perhaps a Riesling, though with a particularly hearty preparation and sauce, reds from Pinot Noir to Merlot to Syrah can work.

Big reds are the unambiguous order of the day for lamb, beef, venison, and sausage. With *lamb,* I like Bordeaux and Bordeaux blends, Merlots, big Pinot Noirs, Rhônes, and Zinfandel. *Beef* invites me to open up those Bordeaux bottles I've been keeping or the big Napa Cabernet Sauvignons. But a

Super Tuscan can be most tempting as well, especially if you've ever had *bistecca fiorentina* (beefsteak). And I challenge you to try Champagne with a grilled steak. It's a real winner. Barbecue also really invites Rhône blends and Zinfandel, which *chez moi* also get the nod for *sausage*. But here's a counterintuitive sausage tip: try a Riesling. *Venison* and anything gamey call for a Rhône or Zinfandel as well, but we favor Pinot Noir.

Other Main Courses

Are wine pairings with spicy ethnic dishes from cultures without winemaking a waste? Some would say so, but I say nonsense. They can in fact provide some of the most beguiling adventures in taste. For *curried fish or chicken* dishes, try a Riesling if you want white or a Zinfandel if red. Hot *Chinese* dishes marry with sparkling wines, as well as Riesling, Pinot Gris, Pinot Blanc, or, for a red choice, Merlot. Spicy *Mexican* goes best with, okay, beer. But try a Riesling, Pinot Gris, or Beaujolais. In my experience, *Thai* often marries well with fruity white wines, Riesling or Gewürztraminer, but also a Pinot Blanc or a sparkling wine. *Couscous?* Red as in Merlot or even a Cabernet Franc or Rhône. *Moussaka?* Merlot, Zinfandel, Sangiovese, or Barbera. *Pizza?* You know I love Champagne, but always think first of a Chianti regardless of the topping. Barbera and Zinfandel are good picks as well.

Cheeses

In the wine business there's a saying: "Buy on apples, sell on cheese." Cheese makes wine look good. Wine and cheese, acid and base, nice marriage. So almost any wine goes with cheese, though some couplings are better than others. Always try local wines with local cheeses. Most people drink reds with cheese, probably because that's what's left in their glass or bottle at the end of a meal when the cheese is served. I belong to the white-wine-with-cheese school and sometimes, though not invariably, switch back to a white for the cheese course after a red wine. So, for *soft goat cheese,* a classic or rosé Champagne, a local white or Sauvignon Blanc, Sancerre, or Chablis; or if you do prefer a red, a Pinot Noir or Merlot. For a *hard goat cheese,* a white Burgundy or Chardonnay; or a Pinot Noir, Merlot, Sangiovese, Syrah, or Cabernet Sauvignon. For a *medium cow's or sheep's milk cheese,* Pinot Noir is my pick. For a *hard cow's or sheep's milk cheese,* Cabernet Sauvignon, Syrah, Merlot, Pinot Noir, Barbaresco, Barolo, or Zinfandel is a good match, but so is a great white Burgundy or Chardonnay or a great rosé Champagne. For *blue and strong cheeses,* sweet wines, such as Sauternes or late-harvest Riesling (*vendange tardive*), Hungarian Tokaji, or Port are ideal.

Desserts

Sometimes a dessert wine *is* dessert. For *apple and other fruit pies* and tarts, try a late-harvest Riesling or a demi-sec sparkling wine. A Sauternes, Tokaji, or *vin santo* might aid and abet your sweet tooth, especially with *berries.* For *melon,* Muscat is great, especially Muscat Beaumes-de-Venise. I don't fancy wine with other fresh fruits or with ice cream. For *creams, custards, and puddings,* many dessert wines work well, from demi-sec sparkling wines to late-harvest Riesling, Muscat, and various ice wines. Those options go for *cakes and cookies,* as would Sauternes, *vin santo,* and Malvasia di Lipari. Finally there is *chocolate.* If you are going to have chocolate for dessert, you really have to decide whether the mouth-filling sweet isn't enough by itself. If not, try a *vin santo* or a Sauternes, a sweet sherry, perhaps a Tokay or Muscat liqueur. And some people like Cabernet Sauvignon. If your last course was with a full-bodied red, you could do worse than to savor the last drops with chocolate.

THE GENTLE ORDER OF THINGS

In the normal course of food-and-wine pairing, we pick what we want to eat and then find a wine to go with it. When the menu is set, we consult a wine list, the sommelier, or a wine merchant for a suggestion. We might also peruse our stash of bottles to see what's on hand and of an age to marry with what we have in mind to eat. Then there are the wine buffs who, as my husband does occasionally, pick the wine first, then the food. Knowing that great food with a bad wine equals a bad experience, and having suffered the pain of enough meals at great restaurants tarnished by a hasty or inappropriate wine choice, he made his own rule. When we dine out at any restaurant for the first time, he starts by reading the wine list, eyeing it for a few "possibilities" he'd enjoy. Then he reads the menu with an eye to finding food that will pair well with the wine or wines he has in mind. The only problem is that often he *reads* the wine list, cover to cover. So when we are dining tête-à-tête, I have to keep up a monologue until he gets his nose out of the *carte.* Oh, well, I'd rather be with someone who cares too much than with one who cares too little. Plus I have my own rule to fall back on: when in doubt, drink Champagne.

7

Thanks to her great cooking, generous spirit, and seemingly limitless energy, my mother was always opening our house to receive others lavishly. It was typically Alsatian of her, but not so typically French. French women may love to outdo themselves once in a while, especially at feasts to mark special occasions like holidays and birthdays, but in general they like to entertain much more than they care to knock themselves out with preparation. They often gather to share some pleasures, but the gathering together is the primary end and the foremost pleasure.

Entertaining is about creating suitable and inviting occasions. It's about bringing people together. This requires the right mix, a group who can enjoy one another's company. But most of all—and here's what we can lose sight of—it is about the guests and not about you. It is about giving and not receiving. I know a lot of people panic or obsess over looking and doing their best. We can all become insecure about hosting and sometimes have the feeling that people are coming to judge us. But that's nonsense. Most of them will have made up their minds about you well before they ever show up; if they've accepted your invitation, that already says a lot. Besides, even reluctant accepters still want to have a good time. Nobody shows up determined not to. Really, you've got them from hello.

So relax. You are who you are. Your home is what it is. Entertaining can be a lot of fun. Just remember to be yourself.

In all cultures, holidays call for particular rituals. People have their expectations, and we don't want to disappoint, so we are inclined to go all out to satisfy, whatever the expectation. It's an expression of love. A dressing of fresh cranberries is surely what the Pilgrims had, if indeed they had anything of the sort, and probably what a foodie would want to serve, but I've met people at Thanksgiving dinners who flip out if not provided with the familiar cranberry aspic that slides out of a can. They don't claim it's better; it's just tradition. (*On ne peut pas plaire à tout le monde:* you can't please everybody.)

Entertaining apart from holidays is a much more liberating experience. It is about bringing people together for its own sake. It is about creating a suitable and inviting occasion on one's own terms. Nevertheless, even such unscripted entertaining is still most of all about the guests and about giving. The choices are perhaps subject to more personal discretion and self-expression, but the key to a pleasant atmosphere (as to overall well-being) is, once again, feeling comfortable in your skin. You don't have to be a domestic goddess to send people home satisfied. In fact, the most ingenious exertions can wind up seeming overconsidered and artificial. *Faites simple*, add touches of your own wit, and all will be well. The seasons, more than any food magazine, should be your guide, with formality—whatever that means to you—being reserved for cooler weather.

Of course, entertaining can have various objectives and therefore different styles: we stage one sort of occasion for a small circle of close friends or relatives, quite another for business colleagues or prospective clients. I do both kinds quite frequently. As a professional in the wine business, I give small dinners as well as orchestrate grand events for hundreds of guests. In our private lives, Edward and I often find ourselves entertaining several times in a week. It's easiest, though generally costlier, to do it at a restaurant. But doing it at home can be simple and inexpensive, no more trouble than making a meal for ourselves, provided we bear in mind the special circumstances of having others in our midst, adding extra touches to distract and delight. And in today's world bringing people into one's home makes a lasting, hospitable impression. Thoughtfulness, not lavishness, is what is appreciated most.

First, there is a matter of self-presentation, which matters to French women. Honor the appearance of guests by giving the appearance of a hostess: dress the part. I don't mean a gown and long gloves; but a slightly more festive top, a more eye-catching bit of jewelry, or some spiffy hostess slippers can show your heart is in the right place. In any case, make sure you're put together. It's awkward to sit down with someone who looks like she's been slaving over a hot stove. For this reason, when entertaining, we put a premium on things that can be made entirely or mostly beforehand and served with a minimum of fuss. It's a question of moderating the experience of your visitors so they don't feel like captives to your attempted hospitality. This feeling usually makes the most jovial guest clam up, which is death to any gathering. But we all have our tricks to promote sociability.

A MOVEABLE FEAST

When it comes to home entertaining, everyone knows you shouldn't keep the guests in one configuration for too long. It slows their circulation, making them listless, and conversational clusters form that never seem to break up. Before you know it, you are entertaining several parties of two or three. There are conventions of mingling, but even these can make an event seem predictable or routine: people generally gather and socialize upon arriving in the living room, move to the kitchen or dining room for the main meal, and perhaps return to the living room for coffee or after-dinner drinks. (Mostly gone are the days when the gentlemen finally repaired to the library for cigars and brandy.) There are, however, less conventional ways to encourage circulation, of both people and their blood.

It's primarily a matter of knowing your space and trying to look at it more imaginatively. If you think of space and area arrangements for a party with a fresh eye, you may find you have more "rooms" inside and perhaps outside than you use. In New York, our apartment has more a vertical than a horizontal configuration. There are three levels inside and two outside. Nice but not as grand as it sounds—remember, this is New York. Think of a small house atop an apartment building. We start the party where the guests are less likely to drift on their own (upstairs) or outside; eventually they find their way back to the more obvious center of gravity, say, in the living room, or somewhere nearer the entrance downstairs, by which time the party is gathering momentum. Further to guest flow, never leave it to the guests to introduce themselves. Whenever one arrives, I walk him or her to another area. If you wind up parking him with another guest, make sure you have given them something to talk about. ("Jean, this is Anne-Marie. She's a great cook; I love her baked ziti." Or "She's just back from a trip to Mexico." What I do not do is introduce people by, or speak about, their professions. French women don't do that. It is ultimately boring and can be awkward.)

Whenever the season permits, we mix indoors with outdoors; going from one to the other is always an agreeable effect, especially in the country. We greet people at the door, lead them to drinks on the terrace, then to another room for dinner. It doesn't have to be where the dining table usually sits. That can sometimes be moved for the occasion. The point is to make the experience seem progressive, not static.

When dinner is promised but time is short, we might move the gathering from home to a restaurant, which can be a wonderful best-of-both-worlds experience. In Paris and in New York, we have a choice of good places a short walk from where we live. (Even more typically in Provence, "Let's get together" means stopping by a neighbor's or friend's house for an apéritif and some nibbles, perhaps meeting some new friends or house guests, then going on to one of the village restaurants.) So we invite the guests to our place for an apéritif: this can be just a glass of Champagne or rosé de Provence and the simplest finger food: olives, melon balls, a few thin slices of salami or prosciutto. The ice is broken, and people are talking, which is harder to achieve when meeting at a restaurant unless everybody knows one another well. You also avoid sitting in a restaurant waiting for your whole party to arrive—nothing less convivial than that (and French people tend to be late). At the restaurant, we go straight to table, often to a main course, which makes the bill less of a bite than it would be for a multicourse dinner. Sometimes we return home again for coffee and dessert. This is the one kind of eating on the go to which I can relate. The pause between courses is there, so nobody eats or drinks too much. It's also a sensible way to balance the expense of eating out with the time commitment of receiving people at home. Plus we've added some walking to the evening. Remember: *La vie est un movement*—literally and figuratively.

CARTE DU JOUR

If you are having people over for a formal dinner, pacing and presenting the experience is everything. Being a good host is not just a matter of what you serve. As in a restaurant, people shouldn't have to sit around twiddling their thumbs wondering what's next. On the other hand, the answer is not to front-load abundance. Your impulse may be to kick things off lavishly with free-flowing spirits and unlimited nibbles, but friends don't let friends eat and drink too much before being seated. (A bunch of groggy adults stuffed with canapés may make for a memorable evening but likely one you would sooner forget.) Consider yourself the manager of everyone's equilibrium for this interval. A drink before dinner does set a tone and can help people relax, but I don't—and suggest you don't—run an open bar before dinner. Offer instead a glass of wine or Champagne. Mineral water should always be offered as well. My mother taught me not to pickle people's taste buds (or your own) before the appreciation of a serious meal and serious cooking effort. (Don't get me wrong, I'm wide open to digestifs and an open bar after the meal, though respecting moderation and balance is at the heart of my philosophy. And remember the 50 Percent Solution: Do you really need [or want] a second single-malt Scotch? Is it as pleasurable as the first? Why not have a glass of water instead—it's good for you.)

As you may recall, anytime I offer wine, I offer food. No exceptions. Among the starters I like to prepare and pass around before a dinner or at a cocktail party are some traditional French ones that I learned from my family.

FINGER FOODS

GEORGIA GOUDA GOUGÈRES

Serves 8

Gougères, little puffs of cheesy choux pastry, are a classic French offering before a meal. (In France, you can buy them in a pastry shop and reheat them, but they are easier to make than your guests will know—and once you get the hang of choux, you can make your own éclairs or profiteroles as well!) They are best eaten warm and so present a bit of a challenge as to timing. Save them for dinners at which the first course won't be served hot. When I was growing up, we had them at home only when Mamie *or someone else in the family could spare the half hour of preparation time before guests arrived. They always appeared when the occasion called for the popping of a cork: Gougères are judged the perfect accompaniment to Champagne. We had dozens of variations in my family, and one aunt (my least favorite, actually) claimed to make the meanest gougères in town. One day, as a sometimes outspoken if not quite rebellious adolescent, I couldn't help jumping into the fray as my mother and my aunts debated the matter. Georgia Gouda Gougères, I declared, were the best! As no one had heard of Georgia, much less her gougères, they had no answer to that.*

I hadn't thought of this experience for decades; then I saw the superb movie Ray, *about the life of Ray Charles. Between the ages of thirteen and seventeen I was a Sunday school teacher, and after class I would meet up with one or two of my best girlfriends, each of us joined by our respective boyfriend* du jour, *to fix Sunday afternoon plans before heading home for the family lunch. We'd rendezvous for twenty minutes at a large and rather ordinary downtown brasserie near the train station, because it had a jukebox full of English and American music. My pal Simone and I had just started studying English in high school, and we enjoyed hearing everything from the Beatles to Sydney Bechet and Ray Charles, though at the time the words were Chinese to us. With incessant repetition, however, we could eventually sing many of the lyrics without knowing the meaning. And as adolescents we were convinced that "Georgia on My Mind" was an ode to a beloved girl, not a place (this despite also having begun to study American geography). The owner's wife used to make gougères for her family's Sunday lunch, and since she liked us, she'd send over a little plate of her minis. Her special touch was to use*

Gouda cheese instead of the more traditional Gruyère. The resulting puffs were great and became our Georgia ("ðgoorðgeeaa") Gouda Gougères, or GGG.

Assuming that I was being adolescent and difficult, my aunts challenged me to produce a recipe. Fortunately, the next Sunday, Madame Lemaire wrote it down for me on a little order slip. I never made them myself back then, but the recipe got high marks from the ladies in my family. My own first attempt wasn't until I was gathering recipes for this book and came across Madame Lemaire's order slip. Standard recipes use milk instead of water and usually Gruyère or Parmesan cheese, not the Dutch Gouda, and they omit shallots and cumin, which may take your guests by surprise.

1. Preheat the oven to 375 degrees.

2. Warm the oil in a frying pan. Add the shallots, and cook over low heat until golden. Let cool.

3. Warm ⅔ cup water in a saucepan, and add the butter and salt. At the boiling point, add the flour all at once, and whisk it with the liquid until a compact, homogenous ball forms. Remove from the heat, and beat in the eggs, one at a time, until the dough is sticky and supple.

4. Add the cooled shallots to dough. Gently incorporate the cheese and cumin seeds.

5. Make small balls of dough with a heaping teaspoon, and place them 1 inch apart on a

INGREDIENTS

1 tablespoon olive oil

2 tablespoons minced shallots

7 tablespoons unsalted butter, cut into small pieces

1 teaspoon salt

1 cup plus 3 tablespoons flour

5 eggs

2 ounces Gouda (or half Gouda, half Comté), diced

½ teaspoon cumin seeds

baking sheet covered with parchment paper. Bake in the pre-heated oven for 20 to 30 minutes, until the puffs are well puffed and golden. Serve lukewarm.

. . . .

QUICHE LORRAINE

Serves 6 to 8

If French women take something as simple as cheese puffs personally, imagine how passions could fly in the province of Lorraine over versions of the namesake quiche. That's one fray I never entered, though I was ever of the opinion that Mother knew best.

Whenever we had guests for lunch on Sunday between fall and Easter, Mamie would give us an early breakfast so she could start her fameux déjeuner du dimanche: *her classic quiche, which can serve as a starter or the single course at a fancy brunch. You could have it with a mixed green salad, unless you prefer to add steamed broccoli or leeks to the quiche batter. Either way, in Alsace, it was well complemented by a glass of the local white or a light red wine. Quiche became quite a rage in the United States a decade or two ago. It got to the point where the claim was being made that real men didn't eat it. But what I found was that men, real or otherwise, and women too, were not having real quiche. The heavy quivering dish often served cold or reheated after sitting for who knows how long in a glass case: this was not the quiche I knew. Here's what real French women eat.*

INGREDIENTS	
1 unbaked pâte brisée, purchased or made from scratch	1. Preheat the oven to 325 degrees.
	2. Roll out the pâte brisée. Line an 8-inch tart pan with the dough, cover it with foil,

fill the foil with dried beans or pie weights, and bake in the preheated oven for 10 minutes.

3. Raise the oven temperature to 375 degrees. Beat the eggs, add the heavy cream and cheese, and season with salt and pepper to taste.

4. Push the bacon into the prebaked crust, and pour in the egg mixture. Bake for 30 to 40 minutes, until set and slightly golden. Serve lukewarm.

INGREDIENTS

4 eggs

½ pint heavy cream or crème fraîche

4 ounces Gruyère or Jarlsberg cheese (or a mixture of both), grated

Salt and freshly ground pepper

3 ounces bacon or pancetta, cubed

· ·

SAINT-JACQUES *TARTINES*

Serves 6

Marraine *Alice, my godmother, was one of those stereotypical French women: thin, chic, with a great sense of style in everything she did, whether it was cooking for the family, entertaining, dressing up, or decorating her home. I spent many vacations during my most impressionable years at her home near Paris. Like my mother, she loved to entertain* (au Champagne s'il vous plaît . . .); *but she had a finer flair for presentation and could set a dazzling table by preparing a few things ahead of time, then adding some plain fresh elements and some store-bought goodies. Her little open-faced sandwiches,* tartines, *are still an inspiration: quartered slices of bread as hors d'oeuvres with bubbly. (Whole slices make a nice lunch.) She thought that conventional sandwiches (with two slices of bread) were too bready (imagine what she would think of our footlong heroes) and unattractive: they hid whatever she had prepared as spread, and looked as good as they tasted. Variety was the key to her magic. There would always be a different kind of bread for each* tartine *and three choices, whether she was making canapés or lunch sandwiches: in spring she favored three fish or seafood choices; in fall and winter it was a trio of meats or cheeses. For lunch, served buffet style (though not all-you-can-eat,* bien sûr*), there was always the accompaniment of a big bowl of mixed salad. Alice believed that six guests were ideal—not so many that she couldn't manage by herself but enough for lively back-and-forth. Her delicious but unpretentiously elegant* tartines *frequently come to the rescue before dinner is served at our house.*

INGREDIENTS

2 teaspoons sherry vinegar

6 mushrooms, cleaned and sliced

10 sea scallops

Salt and freshly ground pepper

4 tablespoons olive oil

1 clove garlic, peeled (if using wooden salad bowl)

4 ounces mesclun

6 slices toasted walnut bread (olive bread is good, too)

1. Pour 1 teaspoon of the vinegar over the mushrooms. Rinse the scallops, pat dry, and season with salt and pepper to taste.

2. Warm 1 tablespoon of the oil in a large frying pan over medium-high heat, and sauté the scallops for 1 minute. Turn over, and sauté 1 minute more. Remove the scallops from pan, and slice.

3. In a bowl (if using a wooden salad bowl, rub it all over with the garlic clove), combine the remaining vinegar and oil. Season with salt and pepper to taste, and toss with the mesclun.

4. Distribute the salad on the toast slices, and garnish with the scallops and mushrooms. Add pepper, and serve.

CRABMEAT *TARTINES*

Serves 6

1. Peel the grapefruit, and separate the slices by taking off the membrane with a knife.

2. Combine the yogurt and paprika. Season with salt and pepper to taste.

3. Distribute the grapefruit and crabmeat on the toast slices. Add some of the yogurt, and serve the rest in a bowl beside the *tartines* so diners can add more if they wish.

INGREDIENTS

1 grapefruit

1 cup yogurt

1 teaspoon paprika or pimento

Salt and freshly ground pepper

8 ounces crabmeat

6 slices toasted fig (or sourdough) bread

GOAT CHEESE AND FENNEL *TARTINES*

Serves 4

Spread the cheese on the bread, top with fennel, season with salt and pepper to taste, and serve.

INGREDIENTS

4 ounces goat cheese

4 slices toasted rye bread

1 fennel bulb, thinly sliced

Salt and freshly ground pepper

LEEK AND SALMON *TARTINES*

Serves 4 hungry people or 8 nibblers

1 sourdough baguette

8 ounces smoked salmon

2 leeks, white parts only,
boiled and sliced

1 tablespoon minced
fresh dill

1. Cut 8 1-inch-thick slices from the baguette.

2. Top each with 1 ounce smoked salmon,
1 tablespoon leeks, and a sprinkling of dill.

OPTIONAL: ADD A FEW DROPS OF FRESHLY SQUEEZED LEMON JUICE OR A DRIZZLE OF

OLIVE OIL.

. . . .

SHRIMP *TARTINES*

Serves 6

INGREDIENTS

1 tablespoon unsalted
butter

2 apples, rinsed, cut into
cubes but unpeeled

Zest and juice of 1 lemon or
lime

Salt and freshly ground
pepper

1 tablespoon olive oil

18 shrimp, peeled and
deveined

6 slices toasted dark bread
(about 2 ounces each)

1. Warm the butter in a large frying pan over
medium heat, and sauté the apple cubes.
Add the lemon juice, and stir for a couple
of minutes. Sprinkle with a bit of lemon
zest and some pepper. Remove the apples
from the pan and set aside. Allow to come
to room temperature before assembling
the *tartines*.

2. In the same pan, warm the oil, and sauté
the shrimp over medium-high heat, stirring frequently. When the shrimp are
cooked, after a couple of minutes, add the
remaining lemon zest and season with salt

to taste. Allow to come to room temperature before assembling the *tartines*.

3. Assemble at the last minute, topping each slice of bread with the shrimp and apples.

. . . .

As to the main event, the key to a sit-down affair is a well-staged sensory experience. It's less what you serve than how you serve it. Any starter/main-course combination I've described that would be suitable for dinner without guests can also be made for company. Inside the family and out, fresh, simple things always satisfy, so long as you have a variety of foods such as one should want for any balanced meal. With company, though, the added frisson of thoughtfulness comes in the presentation, often in the finish. A simple squash purée soup can appear much more dramatic presented with three-inch cuts of chive, like so many pick-up sticks, for pattern and color. For thinner soups you might add some kind of won ton, or homemade croutons. I'm not one for drizzling the plate with zigzags of sauce as some chefs will do. But it is still impor-tant to plate carefully, just as in refined restaurants. The food must look pleasantly arranged, not as if it had been sloshing around on the way from kitchen to table. Family-style serving, though less formal, can be quite appealing, provided it's a dish that looks good in the serving bowl, for instance, beautifully variegated pasta.

Consider the table setting, too: a perfect context to regis-ter the seasons. In summer, especially in the country, I favor a splash of color with lovely place mats, which can be mixed and matched for relaxed fun and a personal touch. In cooler weather, I prefer solids, light or dark, and more tablecloths. Try to vary between place mats and tablecloths—the former for a more modern look, the latter for a more traditional look. In either case, you might consider cloth napkins when you entertain. It's not that much work, and it indicates a place that has been set with care, as does making sure the glasses and flatware are spotless.

Only on the most formal occasions do I fuss about the formality of setting: setting the table with all sorts of specialized cutlery, matching plates for everything, and so on. Usually I prefer to mismatch on purpose. It is more interesting. And no one is going to report you to the police if you serve white wine and red in the same type of glass, or even in the very same glass for that matter. You don't need every piece in your registry to set an elegant table. (Though by all means, if you do buy a complete set of china, make sure it's simple enough to go with different patterns and styles of table linen. Too strong a look can lock you into the same boring table setting for life. And the food on the plate needs to show well.) It can be fun to have a different look of dishware for each course. I like to serve soup in a slightly mismatched set of inexpensive bowls from a pottery shop, followed by a main course on a more conventional plate. If you have more guests than place settings of one china pattern, you could mix two patterns with a certain purposeful symmetry. If the styles don't clash entirely, you can vary the set as you would the guests, alternating boy, girl, boy, girl, and create a great effect. And you can do it with the napkins as well, to reinforce the statement.

A certain fashion has developed around serving small *amuse-bouche* soup portions in demitasse coffee cups, which needn't be made of fine bone china either. Ordinary tableware used unconventionally is one way to be playful and entertaining. Another vessel that I like to conscript for a variety of presentations is the ramekin: It can be used for many things besides *crème brûlée,* from a crab salad to vegetable flan. The portion size is just right for many foods, and don't forget you can get more of them in the dishwasher than you can salad plates. Look at the things you have in your cupboard and use your imagination. If you have little skewers, why not a fruit kebab for dessert instead of a tossed fruit salad? But I'd advise you, don't go overboard with cleverness, and do abandon ideas as they become overexposed, particularly novelties invented by caterers: mashed potatoes in martini glasses were never a good idea.

MORE MOVEABLE FEASTS

The desire to have people over always occurs to me more frequently than my desire to serve them a dinner of several courses. That's a big job: a lot of work, a lot of time, as well as the added expense. The point of entertaining is really just to receive friends in a relaxed setting and make them feel welcome. You can invent occasions to receive them that don't require you to take the day off to cook.

I don't invite people over just for drinks: even with the best of intentions, it encourages alcohol on an empty stomach. And surprise: I'm not the type to dump a bag of chips around a bowl of processed (with corn syrup and worse) dip. But I always offer a choice of finger foods. I do have favorite alternatives, however, which I stage as a sort of open house: the cheese party and the dessert party. Guests are invited to drop by anytime between the hours of x and y. People can come and go, bring children, stay for as little or as long as they care to. The parties require little preparation, so you can socialize with your guests. (I tend to do this both with people I've known forever, just to catch up, and with people I am just getting to know, who might not be entirely at ease or congenial over the course of a long dinner; it's more of a hit-and-run, look-see type of social affair.) If you want to enlarge your social circle, encourage each invitee to bring a friend. One note of caution, however: In France, if someone accepts your invitation, you can expect one in return and are reasonably obliged to accept it. Not everyone in America lives by that rule—thank goodness—or it would be a strong disincentive to entertain. Like my mother, I would rather entertain than be entertained.

Cheese parties and dessert parties are two types of get-togethers I especially like to throw between January and March; on cold Sunday afternoons, they force you out of housebound lethargy and shake off the winter doldrums. If the party is to be held in more than one room, you may want to set up a table or counter in each, varying the selection by room. If you have fewer people or less square footage, setting everything out on one table is fine.

CHEESE-TASTING PARTY

Colette said, "*Un homme qui n'aime pas le fromage ne peut être bien au lit*" (A man who does not like cheese can't be good in bed).

I would say there are probably other liabilities as well. Though it doesn't necessarily follow that French men, cheese lovers to a man, are all great lovers, I will say that the French consider cheese one of the foremost gastronomic pleasures. I'd have to wonder about anyone who didn't like it. Certainly it needn't make you fat, if that's the issue.

French women eat cheese all the time, often instead of dessert. Sometimes they eat both (indulgences) and have a light meal the next time (compensations). I find most Americans like cheese, or at least some cheeses, though they fear it as fattening or artery hardening. First, nothing eaten in proper moderation will make you fat. Second, enjoyed with a bit of wine (see French Paradox, ad nauseam), a moderate amount of cheese is no imminent danger to the cardiovascular system. Besides, I'm suggesting a Sunday afternoon tasting, not a day-long, ten-cheese packdown. A tasting is not a meal; you do it purely for the sensory sensation. If you feel you've thrown your equilibrium off, avoid the stuff for a few days. Reduce your dinner to perhaps just a bowl of soup or some fruit. End of story.

Cheese, of course, is made from cow's milk or goat's milk (sometimes mixed), occasionally ewe's milk, and depending upon aging is soft, medium, or hard. Some cheeses are soft, creamy, and sweet . . . others are hard, smelly, and sharp, and therein lies the adventure of cheese and of the cheese-themed party. There are more than one thousand cheeses made in France alone (as de Gaulle observed, more cheeses than days in the year), but a dozen can make for a full-spectrum tasting party, and as few as six can work fine, too. Some cheeseheads preen like some wine connoisseurs, but don't feel obliged to cultivate comprehensive cheese expertise. I've met a few, and they are the rarest of birds. Ultimately, it's a fool's errand anyway: you could taste and learn about a thousand cheeses, and there would always be a thousand more you haven't tried. (Cheese is made in many more places and ways than wine.) I'm content to live in my world of about a hundred cheeses. I'm always willing to try a new one, but a hundred is more than enough taste reference points for anyone's palate. So, here are just a couple dozen or so winners grouped by relative similarity, none of them unduly hard to find. Some have traditional seasons in which they are best or most readily available. Yes, cheeses have their season (what the animal is feeding on when it delivers milk, like lush summer pastures, and then the optimal aging from that point yield cheese with peak flavors). Otherwise availability is year-round.

Soft Cheeses

- *Brillat-Savarin:* Cow's milk cheese from France, named after the famous gastronome, it is a sharp triple cream with high fat content.
- *Camembert:* Cow's milk cheese from Normandy, but an American artisanal version made in New York or California is a worthy substitute. Soft, creamy, buttery, and mild. You can eat the rind or not. That's a question of taste, but most French people do with this cheese. Good all year. Similar to *Brie* (best November to April) and *Explorateur,* which can have stronger flavors.
- *Fontina:* Cow's milk cheese, from Northern Italy (the soft version is ripe from April to November, the harder,

mature style is best in winter, four months after summer or autumn milk). It has sweet and nutty, sometimes mushroomy, balanced flavors similar to French *Morbier*, and is (relatively) low in fat, and has a telltale ring of ash in the center.

- *Gouda:* A cow's milk cheese from the Netherlands, it is mild and tinted yellow, similar to French *Mimolette*. (But old Gouda is a whole different ball game—strong, more orange, tangy, and nearer to Parmesan in texture and taste.)
- *Mozzarella:* Cow's or buffalo's milk cheese from Italy, it is sweet, milky, and has a slightly resilient texture. California makes good ones. Must be eaten fresh within a couple of days after it is made. It's made all year round, but in spring when made from the milk of cows that graze on sweet, young grass, it can show off an especially floral, grassy, tangy flavor.
- *Robiola:* A mixed-milk cheese from Italy, it is soft and creamy with a mild, earthy flavor. Similar to *Taleggio*.

Hard Cheeses

- *Beaufort:* A cow's milk cheese from France (November to April) that is firm and sweet, with fruit and nut overtones. Wisconsin offers its own version.
- *Cheddar:* A year-round cow's milk cheese from England, it is complex with flavors going from fruity to sharp. Also made in California, Vermont, and many other places.
- *Comté:* An easy-to-like cow's milk cheese from France that's hard but buttery with citrus-like trace flavors.

Like Parmesan, it comes "aged" and develops a wonderful, nutty taste.

- *Manchego:* A sheep's milk cheese from Spain with sweet to nutty flavors and a salty tang.
- *Parmigiano-Reggiano:* A cow's milk cheese from Italy, it is sweet and grassy with fruit overtones.
- *Pecorino:* A sheep's milk cheese from Italy that is strongly flavored with a slightly smoky smell. The best known is *Romano.* It is hard and best for grating, but I fancy small bites of it with a sip of wine.

Blue Cheeses

Penicillium fungus is introduced to create blue veining (part of the gastronomy of decay).

- *Bleu de Bresse:* A cow's milk cheese from France with soft, blue veins, supple and sharp. Similar to the Italian *Gorgonzola.*
- *Fourme d'Ambert:* A cow's milk cheese from France, it is soft, strong with some bitterness and a grainy texture.
- *Roquefort:* A sheep's milk cheese from France that is creamy with spicy and pungent flavors. (Best April to November.) Similar blues of this style are made in the United States, Australia, and England.
- *Stilton:* A cow's milk cheese from England that is a classic, full-flavored blue (Best November to April).

Goat Cheeses

- *Chabichou:* Comes from France and is clean and chalky.
- *Chèvre:* Means *goat* in French and refers to a wide range of soft, semi-hard, and hard goat cheeses that can be set

on bread or added to salads and omelets. A range of good, fresh goat cheeses are made in America.

- *Crottin de Chavignol:* Comes from France and is rather spicy. (Best April to November.)

Extreme Cheeses
(well, that's what some of us call them)

- *Vacherin:* A cow's milk cheese from France that is soft and creamy with a smell of mold and resin and a slightly balsamy taste. Delicious. Cheese lovers go nuts for this woodsy, fruity-flavored cheese over the holidays; best November to mid-April.
- *Époisses:* A cow's milk cheese from France that is soft, rich, strong, and so smelly that I order it only in restaurants, as Edward dislikes it when I keep it in the fridge. It stinks! (Best April to November.) One of my favorites. *Livarot* is even smellier than *Époisses,* and *Muenster,* made in Alsace, is more similar to *Époisses* in taste.

I like to offer cheeses and wines from different countries (though some people prefer to create a spread that is all French, all Italian, all English, or even all American, now that this country has taken a huge interest in cheese that does not come presliced and wrapped in plastic). You can easily get by with a single wine—if so, opt for Champagne, a full-bodied white wine, or perhaps a chilled, dry sherry. If you want things a bit more complex and challenging (at an added cost), select one wine to accompany each individual cheese or grouping. As it is only a tasting, the wine should be poured in very small portions. Put out all the cheese you like, but control the flow from the bottles or you'll have a bacchanal *gratinée* on your hands.

To make the party more of a wine event, you could (1) have a white wine and a red wine; (2) a Champagne, white, red, and sweet dessert wines; or (3) have several whites and reds. Here are some more pairings I like for some of my favorite cheeses:

Soft cheeses: white wines such as Rieslings and sparkling wines. *Hard cheeses:* full-bodied whites, such as Chardonnay; red wines from light to powerful and complex. Goat cheeses go with either whites such as Sancerre, Sauvignon Blanc, or Chablis, and semi to hard goat cheeses also go with lively reds such as Zinfandel or Sangiovese. Blue cheeses pair well with sweet wines, such as Sauternes, or with Port.

Even watching how much you pour, wine-and-cheese parties tend to get louder as the party progresses. So, warn the neighbors. Or better yet, invite them, too.

I like to set out the cheeses garnished with vine leaves, on dark plates (black, bottle green) for contrast. To do it *à la Française,* you'll need some slices of baguette, fresh or toasted; some thick slices of complex seven-grain, olive, or nut breads; or crackers or grissini (fine Italian bread sticks, not Stella D'oro). And only the smallest plates. Finally, not to be nerdy about it, but it helps to put little signs next to each cheese so people take note of what they are tasting as they taste it. If you really want to be obsessive-compulsive, as your guests are leaving, give them a printout of the wines and cheeses served. You don't want a flood of cheese inquiries by phone or e-mail the next day.

Like the cheese-tasting party, this can be as simple or as elaborate as you choose. You can offer as few as four or five desserts, or more than a dozen (careful with those leftovers). You can make your own desserts (I always make at least one or two myself), you can buy them, or you can even turn it into a potluck or a bakeoff. Professionally, I've held dessert parties for which I've brought in pastry chefs from restaurants who set up individual stations at which they served one or two of their specialties. I must say that invite has a nice response rate. For such occasions, I also set up a beverage station with a selection of dessert wines and dessert (demi-sec) Champagnes, but coffee and tea are really all you need, especially in the afternoon.

My selection always includes a lemon dessert (*tarte au citron* is sort of expected from a French woman), something airy like a soufflé (hot or cold), a cake, and a few chocolate desserts (*pots de crème*, mousse, profiteroles), plus a selection of single chocolates from different chocolatiers. When it fits with my travel schedule, I love to bring back a box from a Paris chocolatier like Christian Constant (his ganache cappuccino) and Jean-Paul Hévin (his balao, a caramel ganache in a very dark, slightly bitter chocolate), who do not have stores in New York City. (Alternatively, the Internet provides access to some boutique chocolatiers spread across the United States.) It's the thought that counts (*c'est le geste qui compte*) when the aim is pleasing people.

LAIT DE POULE AU JASMIN

Serves 4 to 6

Here's something that stands out. I can't resist sharing this unusual recipe, as it is a trait of French women to take pride in being a little different, unique in many things. Being "originale" can be exhausting, until you realize that it's okay to take inspiration from others; just put your own spin on their creations. I devised this dessert after seeing it at a restaurant, but that doesn't make it any less of a surprising treat for my guests. Now it can start a little flurry of admiration at your table, too.

A few years ago, we were in Paris when the now famous and impossible-to-book restaurant Astrance (named after a wild mountain flower) opened. Somehow we had learned that both the chef and the manager came from Arpège, one of our favorite star-sprinkled, special-occasion eateries. So we booked a meal at Astrance during its earliest and starless days. And what a meal—easily two stars, we said, our best meal of the year. Four years later, it had indeed won two Michelin stars, putting it in the major leagues of French gastronomy. (And, happily, we are welcomed back like old friends.) The young chef's technique and creativity are astonishing—a signature unlike anyone's I have seen or tasted. L'oeuf (egg) is a case in point. After dessert, half an egg carton is brought to the table. Inside are eggshells with their tops guillotined off, as with oeufs à la coque (soft-boiled eggs). The shells are about half full of a pale yellow liquid that looks a bit like crème anglaise, though somewhat more liquidy. You pick up the eggshells and drink the cool liquid, delicious with a lingering touch of jasmine. That's what I call finger food! It has huge "wow" value, whether at a dessert party or after a good meal. I have adapted the recipe and often serve the eggs in a ceramic egg carton I found in Provence—an object of conversation in itself.

1. Whisk together the egg yolks and sugar until pale and tripled in volume. Add the milk and jasmine tea while continuing to whisk. It should look like a pale yellow cappuccino when done.

2. Serve in empty, prewashed, and dry eggshells.

INGREDIENTS

3 egg yolks

2 tablespoons sugar

1 cup milk (regular or 2 percent)

1 tablespoon cold jasmine tea (rum can also be substituted, as part of the "digestive" notion)

. . . .

CHOCOLATE BRIOCHE

Serves 4

1. Preheat the oven to 325 degrees.

2. Place the brioche slices on a baking sheet and top each with a chocolate bar. Drizzle with 1 tablespoon of the oil, and season with salt to taste.

3. Bake in the preheated oven 4 to 5 minutes, until the chocolate is molten. Drizzle with the remaining teaspoon of oil and serve immediately.

INGREDIENTS

4 1-inch slices of brioche or challah, preferably a day or two old

4 bars (4 squares of 2 ounces each) of dark chocolate (preferably more than 60 percent cacao)

1 tablespoon plus 1 teaspoon olive oil

Sea salt

. . . .

CHOCOLATE *MOELLEUX* WITH WALNUTS

Serves 4

INGREDIENTS

5 ounces dark chocolate
(above 70 percent cacao)

4 tablespoons unsalted
butter, plus more for the
molds

2 eggs, separated

½ cup flour

About ⅔ cup sugar

4 tablespoons fresh walnut
pieces, roughly chopped

1. Preheat the oven to 425 degrees.

2. Break the chocolate into small pieces and melt it with the butter in a bowl set atop simmering water. Let cool, then add the egg yolks and flour. Mix well.

3. Beat the egg whites until they form soft peaks and incorporate in small batches into the melted chocolate. Do the same with the sugar.

4. Butter 4 small individual molds and fill them halfway with the batter. Add 1 tablespoon of walnuts to each mold and cover with more batter. Bake in the preheated oven 12 to 14 minutes, until a crust has begun to form but the middle is still soft. Unmold and serve warm.

CHOCOLATE *PETITS POTS*

Serves 4

1. Melt the chocolate in a bowl set atop simmering water. Add the milk and mix well. Beat in the butter. Pour the batter into small round molds or ramekins.

2. Refrigerate for 2 hours before serving.

INGREDIENTS

7 ounces milk chocolate, coarsely chopped

7 ounces dark chocolate, coarsely chopped

1½ cups milk (regular or 2 percent)

7 tablespoons unsalted butter, at room temperature

. . . .

COFFEE *PETITS POTS*

Serves 4

1. Combine the milk, heavy cream, and sugar in a saucepan. Bring to a boil over medium heat. Add the coffee and beat in the butter. Pour into small round molds or ramekins.

2. Refrigerate for 2 hours before serving.

INGREDIENTS

1 cup milk (regular or 2 percent)

½ cup heavy cream

2 ounces sugar (about ⅓ cup)

2 cold shots strong espresso or ½ cup strong brewed coffee

6 tablespoons unsalted butter, at room temperature

. . . .

PUMPKIN *PETITS POTS*

Serves 4

INGREDIENTS

1 cup milk (regular or
2 percent)

½ cup heavy cream

½ cup pumpkin purée
(canned organic is best)

⅓ cup sugar

1 teaspoon vanilla

¼ teaspoon allspice

6 tablespoons unsalted
butter

2 tablespoons hazelnuts,
roughly chopped

1. Combine the milk, heavy cream, pumpkin purée, sugar, vanilla, and allspice in a saucepan. Bring to a boil over medium heat. Beat in the butter. Pour into small round molds or ramekins.

2. Refrigerate for 2 hours before serving. Sprinkle the hazelnuts on top of each mold just before serving. Toasting the nuts brings out their flavor!

. . . .

LE BRUNCH IS IN

While highly chauvinistic, French women are nevertheless flexible about adopting any foreign influence that suits their overall lifestyle. One of the best inspirations from abroad has been the diversification of breakfast, which is no longer limited to bread, butter, and jam, or croissants. It now extends to cereal and meats, and sometimes even eggs, more like the breakfasts enjoyed in England and America. If only for the introduction of protein in the day's first meal, it's a great leap forward. Apart from yogurt and the classic *café crème* the French breakfast was typically lacking in protein, which is more likely than carbs to sustain one until the next meal.

While I've loved brunch and even featured it at home for all the time I've lived in New York, it is an innovation of the past decade in Paris, where it is now served at home too.

Brunch managed with an eye to portion control—no four-egg omelets followed with a stack of flapjacks to be had à Paris—actually suits the French perfectly: a variety of quality foods enjoyed at a leisurely pace. In some instances, it is even replacing the Sunday family lunch, which can take up half the day. I don't think the French nation could survive the total loss of that tradition—it's especially vital to the social fabric when the family includes kids. But when it's just grown-ups and outside pressures make the long midday meal impossible, *le brunch* can be a nice alternative.

Some of my favorite brunches are admittedly at hotels, among them the Four Seasons in San Francisco (where the ricotta pancakes are a divine indulgence every once in a great while), le Meurice in Paris (where the selection of croissants and Viennoiseries is unmatched), and La Mirande in Avignon (where one could easily linger till mid-afternoon sampling the variety of Provençal specialties such as *fougasses* and other local breads, or lavender honey and jam selections).

But whatever I know about serving brunches at home, I have learned from American women. I remember a fund-raiser hosted by a vivacious lady in Nashville who served an amazing brunch that was more of a fancy *déjeuner sur l'herbe,* her huge backyard flowing with Champagne; her table laden with grits and peach waffles and a gorgeous spinach soufflé. (I had to ask her: "Are you sure you're not French?") I remember another occasion with some Anglophile friends in New England, a chilly fall weekend around a fireplace and lots of scones and clotted cream; there may have even been bangers (everything in moderation). At home in New York, I like to combine French and American touches: farm-fresh eggs from the Union Square Greenmarket, homemade yogurt and oatmeal, fresh croissants and brioches from the local bakery. (If they weren't there, I'd bake the brioches as my mother did. Croissants, on the other hand, are work, but every so often I am stirred to the challenge.) A small glass of just-squeezed orange juice and freshly ground coffee are the beverages, but neither of these quench thirst, so still water is always on the table. Any time the sun shines, even in autumn, though not in the dog days of summer, we serve the brunch on the terrace. Taking our time, the whole thing is done by one o'clock, which leaves a whole afternoon for museums, reading, a little shopping, or perhaps a walk or bike ride. It is the most relaxing way to entertain, and it isn't even French.

COCKTAIL *DINATOIRE*

Halfway between a full-scale dinner production and a theme party, the *∂inatoire* is a very easy and very French way to entertain. It's a sort of dinner buffet, whose name tells guests it's not a sit-down-at-a-dining-room-table affair but more than an apéritif or cocktail in terms of duration and food offerings. *Dinatoire* says you won't leave hungry but advises you not to expect all the formalities of the table. I love the idea, especially during the hectic holiday season when there are so many friends to see and so little time.

The cocktail *∂inatoire* is a most Parisian social gesture, but last Christmas, our friend Marie, a worldly and energetic

Parisienne, hosted one in Provence, reminding me once again that with a little imagination less can most definitely seem like more. Marie bought olives, nuts, and a local baker's puff pastry *petits fours salés* (savory as opposed to the usual sweet ones), which she served with a glass of Champagne. After a lively apéritif hour, "dinner" was served. By then we were all seated in the living room in chairs and couches beside a glowing fireplace, and the food was simply placed on the large coffee table in front of us. As it was holiday time, she had opted to serve smoked salmon and some *foie gras* on toasted brioche, both traditional, accompanied by a glass (or two) of Sauternes. All she had to do was toast the brioche slices, apply the salmon and *foie gras*, and arrange them on a tray. We stayed cozily settled—there was no moving this feast—and ate slowly, relishing the conversation, telling stories, laughing, and meeting new people. No silverware necessary.

The first secret to a successful *cocktail dinatoire* is to pick a good wine: not the most expensive, but not the cheapest; something that shows you've put some thought and care into the choice. The second is the food: A carefully curated menu can make an impression out of proportion to the effort. Prepare your specialty and shop carefully for everything else—or buy everything already prepared and arrange it thoughtfully. A little basket of hard-boiled pretty quail eggs is very little trouble and most inviting. Caviar is a great choice but not within everyone's means or to everyone's taste—a less pricey roe can do nicely. Any artisanal produce could be a good choice: something made and acquired with care. The sweets can be fancy or simple, as you like. Dessert at Marie's was a tray of holiday pastries and cookies. Some people continued with Sauternes, others with coffee or Cognac. Simple, easy, and delicious.

The French have a fancy word for grazing on finger foods: *grignotage.* Nothing new under the sun, really. We owe it all to Spain, the home of tapas, and to Greece, the land of mezze. It's actually a marvelous return to the most elemental satisfactions of eating. Before the fork (which first appeared in the sixteenth century), we all ate with our fingers. *Grignotage* is perfect for an age in which time is shorter and caloric requirements are not what they were when we labored in the fields from sunup to sundown. A *cocktail dinatoire* is also time elastic, from, say, as little as two hours' duration to the hours and hours of a traditional French dinner.

The small morsels of the *cocktail dinatoire* are certainly in line with the French woman's notion of eating *menu* servings (the French use the word in the sense of an order of little things to be served, not in our sense of a list of options). But this "new" old habit of eating a series of small bites also serves the necessity of taste and variety when the pace of life has made the long leisurely meal more and more the exception than the rule. The French can't all sit down every evening for a longer dinner, much as they continue to relish the custom when they can. In the past thirty years, the average French meal has been reduced to about thirty-four to thirty-six minutes, a third of what it was before (yet this is substantially greater than the American average meal of twelve to sixteen minutes, often consumed while doing something else as well). Abbreviated though it has become, eating in France is not yet a grim and rushed affair. Under the new constraints the French still do not attempt to cram two hours' worth of eating into thirty-six minutes. That interval is simply not sufficient for eating a meal of several full courses properly. Rather than eat faster, the French choose to eat less in the time allotted them. And they are not in danger of starving. They know a shorter menu of high-quality, varied foods can satisfy both the senses and the body's nutritional demands. As I've noted, it takes only twenty minutes of slow, mindful eating for the brain to signal the end of hunger. If the food is good and we are concentrating on its pleasures, healthful satisfaction is still possible.

FINAL TIP

Sometimes entertaining seems like something we hate doing but love having done. The extra work and a little gratuitous anxiety over things that could go wrong can always present enough of an excuse not to bother. When in doubt, ask yourself—as my mother taught me to do—what's the worst thing that can happen? The cake doesn't rise, wine gets spilled, a guest is rude, the bill is steep, you have to get up an hour earlier, the dog eats your *foie gras*? All relatively minor. Life goes on. Chances are, things will go well, people will have a good time, and you'll feel good about it for some time to come. So go for it. Though it's all about giving, you really do get back more than you give.

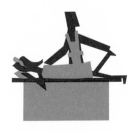

À BIENTÔT:

A LITTLE FRENCH LESSON

Languages have always been one of my special interests, and I find there is no quicker way to get into a culture than to absorb a bit of its language. Even words that have the same definition in one language can have a very different connotation or nuance in another. And connotation and nuance, that sense of words beyond the totally literal, is where the essence of culture resides. It differentiates even two cultures that supposedly speak the same tongue. As George Bernard Shaw said, "England and America are two countries separated by a common language." Imagine how much a totally different language estranges us from the French.

I obviously believe there are valuable things to be learned from traditional French living. As I have said, a lifestyle is more than a list of habits in isolation; it's a total mind-set and in this case a culture. So if you want to live a bit like a traditional French woman—training yourself to tune in to peak sensory experience, to live in the season, to eat for pleasure and not get fat—being able to get inside the "head" of French culture is a big help.

My first professional training was as a translator-interpreter. I remember one translation class at my university in which we had to learn the rules of cricket. For a French girl, this was as alien as studying a repair manual for a spaceship. We never got to American baseball (I doubt the professor understood it), but the point was that any important part of a culture, in this case sports, infiltrates the language and provides its metaphors. Living in the United States, I appreciate how important baseball is to our American language and culture. I've been to enough games to know what a home run is. (That's when your hotel room isn't ready and they upgrade you to an available suite with an ocean-view terrace, right?) Anyway, the language of whatever preoccupies a people—be it their food, fashion, lifestyle, the arts, sports, even business—is a unique window on their being.

The French are inordinately proud and protective of their language, which for a millennium was the world's language of diplomacy and for centuries the lingua franca for style, fashion, and many of the arts. There is even an official body, the Académie Française, a collection of forty writers, artists, academicians, and politicians (called the *Immortels*) who meet on Thursday afternoons to rule on what's correct language usage and what isn't. (An inconceivable notion in America, where usage seems to morph at the speed of streaming video.) It is a source of continuing pride and wonder that even today in America far more students are studying French than Chinese, Russian, or Arabic, say—languages whose knowledge may seem more vital to our future. In any case, you don't have to learn the language fluently to absorb the lifestyle. As with French portions, a little can go a long way, if you choose well.

In that spirit, here's a little French vocabulary list *à ma façon* useful for all seasons. It is drawn chiefly from words and concepts I have used in this book. Alas, there are no sports metaphors.

Bien dans sa peau [byeh(n) dah(n) sah poh]: Healthy French women achieve the state of being "comfortable in one's skin." For all her attention to what she wears and what she eats, a French woman is most defined by her ease in being herself and the attractiveness that comes of relishing her pleasures. French women achieve this state more intuitively than most, but not everyone is successful. The secret of the woman who continues to be *bien dans sa peau* is that she has come to terms with enjoying each phase of her life and adjusting to life's different seasons. Being comfortable with oneself is such an important concept that I want to share another illustration, *une petite histoire*.

Every year we go back to Paris for the year-end holiday season when the Christmas decorations are low-key but lovely and the museums tend to be less crowded and so much more enjoyable. One of our little traditions is that Olivier, who is an inimitable art *conférencier* and the brother-in-law of a friend, gathers a dozen of us at the Musée du Luxembourg at the Sénat to comment on the current art exhibition. In late 2005 and early 2006 we saw the splendid Phillips Collection (Washington, D.C.) of French art from the nineteenth and twentieth centuries. The group attending varies slightly from year to year as some of us can't always make it. For me, it's one of those small pleasures not to be missed. Among the newcomers that year were two women over age fifty. One, Edith, was stunning: slim, full of energy but gently so, with a great haircut, a simple, long black coat, very little makeup, a sense of self-confidence, and emanating an air of serenity and *douceur de vivre*. Her age didn't really matter. She had that *je ne sais quoi* of the mythical French woman. She had adjusted well to time and age.

The other, Claudine, was a bit plump, didn't quite look as though she was *bien dans sa peau,* and in her conversation didn't sound as if she was. She vaguely offered what I believe, that at around fifty, women have to start making choices such as cutting down on food and wine portions, increasing the number of walks and whatever exercise we do, drinking more water, getting enough sleep, and, most important, picking our indulgences . . . but also wearing less and different makeup, deciding what to do about hair color and style, and giving up certain clothes. In other words, to some extent we have to reinvent ourselves for the next season of life. Claudine knew that but didn't practice it. Being comfortable in one's skin is not simply a question of slim versus plump. Edith, however, knew that this season in life is also often a time for new friends, perhaps some new hobbies; the main point is to remain active, curious, enthusiastic, and optimistic. The most positive among us, like Edith, do it almost effortlessly as if one more challenge is welcome. The feeling of well-being is ever so crucial in the way we age and confront the later phases of our life. No *laissez-faire*. No *laissez-aller*.

Bio [bee-OH]: In their pursuit of quality over quantity French women increasingly select organic (or as they call them, *bio* foods) at markets and shops. Whether organic foods are more nutritious than regular foods is debatable; they are at least as nutritious, but for about the same price—sometimes a bit more, occasionally a bit less if they are local—they spare us ingesting chemical fertilizers and pesticides. And, of course, they are superior to processed foods. *Bio* is as fast a developing market in France as it is in America. But the French are a bit more skeptical about labels; they know that "organic" can mean different things to different governing authorities. If "organic" becomes just a marketing strategy, supply will have to expand to compete with demand, and standards may suffer. That's why we always prefer foods that taste as they were meant to taste. For that, local producers, who are more likely to grow organically, and whose offerings are more likely to be fresh and seasonal, are more reliable than labels. Organic is a good thing but only if we keep it real.

Bonheur [boh(n)-UHR]: French women know happiness is not a matter of luck; it's what you make of your life. This word for happiness is literally "good time." The French way of connecting feeling with time is telling. It suggests something to be cultivated in the course of our hours and days and months and years, how we live in relation to them. The English word *happy* comes from the archaic word *hap*, which means "luck." Interesting distinction.

Bonjour [BOH(N)-zhoor]: A French woman's first word to anyone, be they stranger or friend, is usually *bonjour*: good (*bon*) day (*jour*). The salutation is at the heart of French culture and etiquette, and if you listen the emphasis is almost always on the good side: BON-jour. If you are the sixty-eighth person of the day walking into a small shop, you will be greeted with *bonjour* as were the previous sixty-seven and as will be the sixty-eight who follow. It's an ingrained social ritual, and you must return the store clerk's *bonjour* before anything else, such as asking a question. In New York, complete sentences, let alone verbal niceties, can seem a waste of time to most. (On the other side of the world, credit goes to the Australians who have kept up G'day in a positive spirit.) In France, where the relation to time is different from America, not to observe these customs is considered rude. You have a much better chance of being treated nicely if you say *bonjour* to everyone you meet. If it is evening, *bonjour* becomes *bonsoir*. "Good evening." Only friends use the word *salut*, "hi" and "bye." The farewell matters, too. When you leave a store, don't be surprised if the clerk says good-bye, even if she is occupied with another customer. You should not neglect to say, *"au revoir"* ("good-bye" but more literally, "until we see each other again: time again") and always *"merci."* Among friends we also say *à bientôt* ("see you soon"). These pleasant little expressions go a long way in France to help people connect in a friendly and effective manner.

Bricolage [bree-koh-LAZH]: French women (and men) have made an art of making do with what's at hand, whether with one's clothes, or what's in season at the market, or available in a storeroom or closet. When I removed a mirror from a wall not long ago, exposing an embedded hook, I had to figure out what to do about that eyesore. I discovered a long-forgotten, old ceramic "art" plate that I had bought years ago but had never found the right place to hang. Now I did, though it was never intended for this sort of wall covering. The ceramic is not the *Mona Lisa,* but guests are repeatedly drawn to it. It covers a blemish as if it were born for that spot and gives the room a fresh, distinctive, and harmonious look.

I love this word, *bricolage,* which comes from the verb *bricoler,* to tinker about, mostly around the house. Though implying somewhat mechanical applications (there's a chain of hardware stores in France called Mr. Bricolage), the word certainly has an extended definition covering how one combines things in the kitchen or even how one puts oneself together in clothes. It has special cultural meaning in that it celebrates a person, *un bricoleur* (masculine) or *une bricoleuse* (feminine), who is creative and imaginative and who puts things in fresh and original ways. Recently nine out of ten French women admitted to adoring *bricoler.* A friend, for instance, recently made a celebratory, nonedible, birthday cake for her eight-year-old out of flowers from her garden. When I go to the market and the eggplants are in season, I tend to overbuy to capture the moment to the fullest; I come home and then have to figure out how to incorporate them variously into our meals over the next few days. Ratatouille, for certain, but what about using the barbecue to grill them or the vegetable mill to purée them into a spread to start lunch or dinner? Once I went fishing off Long Island and came home with forty-eight mackerels, but that's another story. Sometimes I get really creative and think I've invented a new dish, only to find it on a restaurant menu later. Good chefs are great *bricoleurs*.

Une certaine tenue [ewn sehr-TEHN ten-EW]: A French woman expresses her indefinable flair through that certain something, an added element. It's said we know how to *jouer l'accessoire* (to accessorize). And it's true, the French woman's style has much to do with this knack. But it's not so much the accessories themselves; rather the choice of this (rather than that) as a form of self-expression. As with so many things, less is more. One element—a handbag, a bracelet, even a lipstick—can pull a look together, making it *bien tenu*. Mixing elements, for example, something precious with an item bought from a street vendor, is what stylists and designers do. French women do it for themselves, adding a touch that is entirely individual—sometimes witty and idiosyncratic, perhaps even a little eccentric, but not tacky. It's all about knowing themselves well enough to make the choice self-expressive: this is the French woman's edge.

C'est la vie [seh lah vee]: French women know there is a certain serenity in knowing those things you can change from those things you can't, and French women strive to know the difference. When they use the expression "that's life," it expresses an acceptance, even an embrace, of those things we cannot change, such as getting older and the rhythm of the seasons. But it is also accepting little things. I know when I am in France and at a post office that closes at 5 p.m. and the clerk stops selling stamps ten minutes early (to pack up, of course) or when I show up at the hairdresser for my appointment for a blow-dry and the smiling and chatty *coiffeuse* is an hour behind,

I have to tell my American self to stop and think, *"c'est la vie"* (or sometimes, *"c'est la France"*).

Champagne [shahm-PAH-nyuh]: A French woman's eyes sparkle when she hears the word, and even more when she's offered a glass. She will always answer—and here I speak from extensive experience—*"volontiers"* ("gladly," but literally, "most willingly"). Champagne is a state of mind, a very pleasant one. It is made in the Champagne region of France and serves as a mood enhancer the world over. It is at once history and culture and pleasure and celebration, quality and refinement. The sound of a cork popping is magic.

Embracing Champagne as part of French culture starts young in France. Some people in France place a drop on their infant's forehead or behind his or her ears when christened. My first memory of drinking the real thing was when I was six. Recently I had the pleasure of dining at a top French restaurant with a group of six- and seven-year-olds as part of an educational enrichment program. They all started the meal nonchalantly with a glass of bubbly. I was taken aback for a moment, but then asked a little girl if she liked Champagne, and she said, "It is Champagne d'Enfant, Madame." (Children's Champagne.) The bottle was the same, the label looked just like one on a Champagne bottle, the pop was the same, the glass used was the same as I had for my Champagne, and the bubbles were lively, but the bubbly was nonalcoholic apple cider. It seems these kids always celebrate their birthdays and special occasions with Champagne d'Enfant.

Détox [day-TOX]: French women are very mindful of the process of flushing out the waste products of metabolism that reside in our tissues, aiding our liver in its constant detoxing of our bodies. It's not just hedonism, for example, that makes French women love massages, and it's not only for the tactile pleasure. The vigorous touch of another can stimulate the lymphatic system, loosening stagnant toxins. For this reason, after a massage one is always offered a glass of water. While getting the toxins moving is one thing, nothing flushes them out like the process by which we absorb and eliminate water—again a reason to hydrate plentifully after a massage. And in today's world of preservatives, pesticides, artificial colors, flavors, and sweeteners, we have a lot to flush. The occasional Magical Leek Soup weekend is also as good a detox regimen as you'll find at any spa. (I appreciate professional massages can be expensive, but it's something partners can easily learn to do for each other.)

Eau [oh]: This French woman begins each day with a glass of water and makes sure to have a glass just before going to bed. Water is mythically one of the basic elements, along with fire, air, and earth. It is so vital to the French they denote it with a single vowel sound. French women drink it all day long. It is essential for every bodily process. We absorb it in some of our foods: soup is rich in water and it's known that a meal started with soup is one in which we will typically eat less overall. Some beverages are mostly water, but there is only one way to get enough: drink water itself. And drink it for the taste. (Too many people lose the taste for water by preferring to drink anything but. The idea that a meal might taste better with a diet soda than a glass of water is utterly alien to French women.) Hydration plumps tissue but not with fat. Learning to hold more water not only makes all our bodily processes work better, it also leaves skin clearer and fuller. There is never a time of year not to drink plenty. We lose 80 ounces a day in respiration alone. But in extreme heat and cold, hydration requires more vigilance. As you practice increasing your water intake steadily throughout the day—think six- or eight-ounce glasses—your body becomes more efficient at making use of what it was hoarding before. Just see what drinking water does for your breath. Now there are times when I compensate for all the added water by eating a few mildly diuretic foods: leeks, asparagus, cherries, grapes. Stronger diuretics, like any drink with alcohol or caffeine, need to be taken in moderation since they dehydrate and stimulate appetite. Finally, remember that some experiences of hunger are only thirst in disguise. So try answering the sensation with water first.

Entre deux âges [AHN-truh douze ahzh]: **French women have a** phase in life, literally "between two ages," or of ambiguous age. To be able to appear so is one of the advantages of living like a French woman. Nothing can alter the fact of the number of years you have lived, and some changes with time are inevitable. But how quickly the body ages depends in large part on how you take care of it, especially on what you put into it and whether you keep it moving throughout the day, every month of the year. Aging gracefully, French women don't suffer the ravages of time too fast, and so they learn to be comfortable with their age. It's an important element of living *bien dans sa peau,* which is the key to feeling good and being attractive. You don't have to be old to be a *grande dame* . . . just great.

Équilibre [eh-kee-LEEBR]: **French women know that main-**taining balance or a healthy equilibrium is all-important and takes work, though after a while it becomes a continuous, unconscious activity. In terms of food, the notion of equilibrium as it pertains to living like a French woman is the balance between the calories one consumes and those one expends exerting oneself. French women don't aim to "burn" calories. They eat to fuel their bodies in proportion. If they overeat they don't plan to balance by overexerting themselves later. (If they overindulge, they simply eat less later.) Walking and the more intense routine exertion of taking the stairs are the French *équilibristes* secret agents.

Equilibrium is maintained in several time frames: daily (*quotidien*) balance is, for example, if you have a big fancy dinner, you have a soup or salad for lunch the next day or go for a walk after supper. If you can't square the books the next day, do so by the end of the week. The balance for maintaining weight is weekly (*hebdomadaire*). The yearly equilibrium (*équilibre annuel*) is maintained by observance of the seasons.

But what of the monthly (*mensuel*)? For a stretch of our lives many of us face an added equilibrium challenge. (To some, it can seem a month-long affair every month, from premenstrual syndrome to menstruation to postmenstrual syndrome.) The difficulty of the experience varies by individual, but French women have traditionally done a few things to ease the symptoms. First, avoid too many carbohydrates at breakfast. Replace orange juice and other sugary things with a bit of protein, such as slivers of boiled ham or prosciutto and a small piece of cheese. For me, yogurt has always been a life-saver, especially when I had more than one a day to ease cramps and control cravings. And something a little counterintuitive: although you may be feeling bloated, do not neglect hydration. Try a big glass of lukewarm water (it's easier to absorb) with a squeeze of lemon first thing when you get up. When you are retaining water, the best way to get rid of it is to add more.

Faites simple [feht sahmpl]: French women know that generally less is more and when you start with quality—keep it simple. In terms of food, "simple" means less preparation and cooking time required, especially when you use marvelously fresh food. In terms of wardrobe, French women are likely to have only a few prime garments per season, but they are quality pieces that can be handsomely dressed up or down with the use of accessories, making it easier to put yourself together.

Joie de vivre [zhwah duh VEEV-ruh]: French women know that a healthy mind and body, taking pleasure in the seasons and in things great and small, are all part of "the joy of living," joie de vivre (an expression for which there is sadly no American equivalent). One sure way to maximize your joie de vivre is to become a student of *l'art de vivre,* cultivating an appreciation of balance and gratification in all forms of sensory experience.

Laissez-aller [LEH-say al-LAY]: French women rarely give up on themselves, literally, to let oneself go. They know that it's never too late to be beautiful and that being beautiful is nothing more than maintaining themselves physically and mentally at any given interval of life. Coco Chanel said, "Nature gives you the face you have at twenty, life shapes the face you have at thirty, but at fifty you get the face you deserve." The fashion industry would like to make us think that a fifteen-year-old girl is the ideal of beauty. Subtext: After that, what's the point? I'm amazed to find lovely young thirty-year-olds in New York who consider themselves past it. Sometimes they make the mistake of trying to seem younger in clothes and styling, but ironically when one appears to be hiding one's years, one only winds up seeming older. Then there's being *figée* (unevolving, frozen) and *coincée* (uptight: we age but our presentation stays the same, for instance keeping the same hairstyle for ten years). French women do make the most of themselves at every age, and it's a matter of adaptation—it's up to each of us to construe our own beauty. They believe in *beauté charme:* the total effect beyond just a nice body and a pretty face; it includes the way one talks, smiles, moves, and gestures. If we are confident in feeling energy, depth, and charisma, we naturally transmit the feeling with our body and face. Beauty and its seductiveness are generated from within, not applied from without. As the fox in Saint-Exupéry's *Little Prince* says, "One sees the essential only with the heart. The essential is invisible to the eyes."

La Moitié [lah MWAH-tyay]: When being served meat, vegetables, soup, whatever at someone's home or even in a restaurant, French women are apt to tell the person dishing it out, *"la moitié, s'il vous plait"*: just give me half of that. It's mainly rhetorical in a French setting, where you are far less likely to get an outsize portion. But in other places, it's a survival tactic. This is the 50 Percent Solution in practice. How much do you want to eat? How much should you eat? How about half?

Nos petits démons [noh puh-TEE day-MOH(N)]: French women, indeed all women, have their little demons, their personal offenders. They can be foods whose siren song is most likely to mess up our equilibrium. The only answer to their danger is to identify them and to enjoy them with extra care. None should be forbidden; your discipline is not to skip them but to practice eating them mindfully and with focus. For those who are inclined to empty a bag of nuts, for instance, it is an excellent mental yoga practice to eat one nut at a time, up to five, very slowly, until you get to the point where it's simply too boring to contemplate having another one (shelling your own helps in this discipline).

Apart from chronic offenders we must also be on guard for cravings, especially at the most hormonally turbulent time of the month. I often answer cravings with a bit of dried fruit, such as figs, apricots, or prunes. Another excellent answer to this faux hunger are the French gherkins, or *cornichons*. Something about the vinegar and spice of these little pickles and their intense hit of flavor tends to dispel cravings. I find this is true of licorice as well, a fresh, intense taste that somehow turns off your desire to eat.

I confess to chocolate and bread as two of my demons (not-so-uncommon personal offenders), but happily, shopping is not a third. *Nos petits démons* are not limited to food. I don't binge on new shoes or clothes as a pick-me-up (keeping the same size and weight since adulthood helps). But the drill is the same. Know your offenders and indulge mindfully and in moderation in order to maintain equilibrium. And if once in a while you succumb to your demons? Congratulations: You are human. Forget the guilt and remember to compensate over time to regain your balance.

Petits riens [puh-TEE ryeh(n)]: French women love their little nothings. A misnomer, really, and all a matter of perception. I love the $5 and $10 gifts I receive, incalculably great and incalculably small. It could be a candle, a flower, four chocolates, a nifty magnet for the refrigerator with a clever phrase or picture, a ceramic insect (I did not think that was possible until I got one). In a complex world we have conditioned ourselves not to sweat the small stuff. It's true, you shouldn't sweat small things, but you should enjoy them. I am not speaking of the little irritations we face but about things that seem incidental but can enhance experience and give pleasure. When it comes to our *petits riens* we don't need to know exactly what they add to the fullness of our experience; we need only to be open to the possibility that seeming trivialities may play a significant role in how we feel overall.

Peu à peu [puh ah puh]: French women appreciate that Rome wasn't built in a day (and neither was France), but rather "little by little." The progress of your life toward peak experiences in all aspects of living will take time. Changes made drastically or all at once are often the sorts of modifications that don't stick. Like New Year's resolutions, they are upheld proudly for a little while, but then we fall back to our old ways. Arrive at your new ways gradually, and you will leave your old ways too far behind for easy return. And if you slip up a bit, you won't feel a failure; you will know how to get back on track because it isn't all or nothing. It's a game of inches.

Plage de temps [plahzh duh tahm(p)]: French women are hedonists without being narcissists, but also pragmatists who understand that a healthy balance of pleasure in life requires a "beach of time," a lovely expression meaning a space of time for oneself to which one repairs on a daily or periodic basis. Sometimes it means making a morning for oneself—I have had to make a practice of scheduling a beach day for myself— or sometimes it can be a half hour or just a few minutes. It can be found in the most unlikely places: when you are stuck in traffic, listening to music, or just doing routine chores. You can let your mind fill up with anxiety or resentments, or with a bit of practice you can learn to head to the beach. The mind is its own place.

De saison [duh say-ZOH(N)]: French women know life would be tedious if it came in only one flavor. Whether fashion, food, or travel, French women anticipate and indulge in what's "in season." It's fun to be *"au courant"* with respect to the latest in food, drink, style. But this does not mean we don't pay proper attention to *les classiques,* whether they be the little black dress or the best of foods that return and give indispensable pleasure year after year. Alas, to define *de saison* properly takes a book (hopefully this one).

Terroir [tare-RWAHR]: French women know it is a combination of soil, sun, and microclimate that makes the same variety of melon from farmer Chassain taste sweeter than that from farmer Dubois. I am mindful of this when I shop locally at the Union Square Greenmarket, where I can choose tomatoes or strawberries from a half dozen vendors, but always seek out the one whose fruit is to my taste. The cultivation of the *terre* (soil, earth) and seasonal weather also have a big impact on quality, which is why wine vintages can vary so much in quality and characteristics from year to year, and from producer to producer, but it all starts with the *terroir*, which imparts distinctive quality to what is cultivated locally on the spot. *Terroir* is virtually a holy word in the world of wine, whether in Alsace, Champagne, Bordeaux, or elsewhere, but especially in Burgundy, vines planted six feet apart can produce grapes and then wines that are unmistakably different in character and often quality as well. This difference—validated over centuries of harvests—is always registered in the price, sometimes in multiples of five or more from vineyard to vineyard. There is a group of oenophiles who are such militant followers of *terroir* they call themselves "*terroiristes*."

Les vacances [lay vah-KAH(N)s]: French women take their vacation, *les vacances*, very seriously. The French motto is liberty, equality, brotherhood (*Liberté, Egalité, Fraternité*), but along with these inalienable rights, the French add six weeks of vacation. *Bien sûr*. It is a subject and measure of time that shapes their year. Implicit is the deep belief in the need to recharge one's batteries and that self-indulgent "play" is a psychological necessity to well-being. Vacations are so institutionalized in France that the majority of the *citoyens* (citizens) take them at the same time. It used to be that for the entire month of August the highways leading from Paris had nonstop traffic alerts and long delays. Some years ago the government "asked" large companies to encourage some vacations starting on July 1 or July 15 to keep the economy and traffic flowing, but August is still pretty congested. The winter vacations are fixed by the national school calendar. And I continue to be amazed by how many French people still take their vacations exclusively in France. What's not amazing, in fact it's quite common, is to hear French people on vacation talking about their next vacation.

En vélo [ah(n) vay-LOH]: French women are much more likely to travel *en vélo*, "by bike," than Americans, but as in China the days of bicycles being a primary means of transportation are greatly diminished. However, French women are terrific at incorporating bursts of physical activity as part of their daily routine (as opposed to going to the gym)—walking, of course, taking the stairs, even swimming when possible. Today bicycling is still a top recreational activity in France. Go to a sporting goods store and see all the special clothing and accessories and varieties of bicycles in all sizes and prices. It seems everyone lives Le Tour de France (and dresses the part). When I am out for a scenic ride and am huffing and puffing up some gradual climb with my mind on vacation, I am sometimes awakened by the sound in my left ear of the word "*bonjour*," a signal I am about to be passed by some man or woman or *peloton* (pack) on their racing bikes speeding on their way.

Voilà [vwah-LAH]: This is what French women (and men) say when all is said and done, and the thing speaks for itself: here it is, voilà, the end of *French Women for All Seasons*. I hope you enjoyed it and benefited from it. And I hope it speaks for itself.

Bonne chance et bonne continuation.